# AIR FRYER RECIPES

### 300

## This Book Includes : "Air Fryer Cookbook + The Affordable Air Fryer Cookbook + The Air Fryer Recipes "

By Denise White

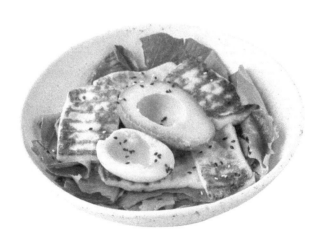

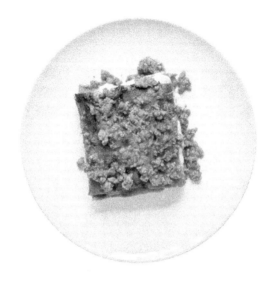

# AIR FRYER COOKBOOK

Table of Contents

Introduction 19

Air Fryer Recipes 21

1. Squash Oat Muffins 21

2. Hash brown Casserole 24

3. Mexican Breakfast Frittata 24

4. Perfect Brunch Baked Eggs 25

5. Green Chile Cheese Egg Casserole 26

6. Kale Zucchini Bake 28

7. Cheesy Breakfast Casserole 29

8. Easy Hash Brown Breakfast Bake 31

9. Mexican Chiles Breakfast Bake 31

10. Delicious Amish Baked Oatmeal 32

11. Pork Sirloin Steak 33

12. Chicken Meatballs with Cream Sauce and Cauliflower 35

13. Shrimp Salad 36

14. Maple Asparagus Salad with Pecans 38

15. Creamed Kale 39

16. Baked Zucchini 39

17. Roasted Broccoli Avocado Soup 40

18. Herbed Tuna 42

19. Sirloin Steak 42

20. Whole Chicken 43

21. Mini Sweet Pepper Poppers 44

22. Spicy Spinach Artichoke Dip 44

23. Personal Mozzarella Pizza Crust 45

24. Garlic Cheese Bread 46

25. Crustless Three-Meat Pizza 46

26. Smoky BBQ Roasted Almonds 47

27. Beef Jerky 48

28. Pork Rind Nachos 48

29. Ranch Roasted Almonds 49

30. Loaded Roasted Broccoli 50

31. Scrumptious Leg of Lamb 51

32. Chinese Style Pork Chops 51

33. Cinco De Mayo Pork Taquitos 52

34. Tangy Smoked Pork Chops with Raspberry Sauce 53

35. Air fryer toast oven bacon 54

36. Italian Pork Milanese 55

37. Jamaican Jerk Pork Roast 56

38. Tasty and Moist Air Fryer Toast Oven Meatloaf 57

39. Classic Country Fried Steak 59

40. Bourbon Infused Bacon Burger 60

41. Glazed Lamb Chops 62

42. Buttered Leg of Lamb 63

43. Glazed Lamb Meatballs 64

44. Oregano Lamb Chops 65

45. Lamb Steaks with Fresh Mint and Potatoes 66

46. Lamb Kofta 66

47. Crunchy Cashew Lamb Rack 67

**48.**Oregano & Thyme Lamb Chops *68*

**49.**Lamb Meatballs *69*

**50.**Thyme Lamb Chops with Asparagus *69*

**51.**Cornflakes French toast *70*

**52.**Mint Galette *71*

**53.**Cottage Cheese Sticks *71*

**54.**Palak Galette *73*

**55.**Spinach Pie *73*

**56.**Balsamic Artichokes *74*

**57.**Cheesy Artichokes *75*

**58.**Artichokes and Special Sauce *76*

**59.**Beet Salad and Parsley Dressing *76*

**60.**Beets and Blue Cheese Salad *77*

61.Shrimp Pancakes *78*

62.Shrimps with Palmito *78*

63.Gratinated Pawns with Cheese *79*

64.Air fryer Crab *80*

65.Crab Balls *81*

66.Crab Empanada *82*

67.Crab Meat on Cabbage *83*

68.Gratinated Cod *83*

69.Gratinated Cod with Vegetables *85*

70.Salmon Fillet *86*

71.Hake Fillet with Potatoes *87*

**72.**Delicious Raspberry Cobbler *88*

**73.**Orange Almond Muffins *89*

**74.**Easy Almond Butter Pumpkin Spice Cookies *90*

**75.**Moist Pound Cake *91*

76.Banana Butter Brownie *92*

77.Peanut Butter Muffins *92*

78.Baked Apple Slices *93*

79.Vanilla Peanut Butter Cake *94*

80.Moist Chocolate Brownies *95*

81.Yummy Scalloped Pineapple *96*

82.Vanilla Lemon Cupcakes *96*

83.Walnut Carrot Cake *97*

84.Baked Peaches *98*

85.Cinnamon Apple Crisp *99*

86.Apple Cake *100*

87.Almond Cranberry Muffins *101*

88.Vanilla Butter Cake *102*

89.Coconut Butter Apple Bars *102*

90.Easy Blueberry Muffins *103*

91.Tasty Almond Macaroons *104*

92.Moist Baked Donuts *105*

93.Eggless Brownies *105*

94.Vanilla Banana Brownies *106*

95.Choco Cookies *107*

96.Chocolate Chip Cookies *108*

97.Oatmeal Cake *109*

98.Delicious Banana Cake *110*

99.Chocolate Cake *111*

100.Almond Blueberry Bars *112*

Conclusion 114

# THE AFFORDABLE AIR FRYER COOKBOOK

## Table of Contents

Introduction..................................................................................119

Air Fryer Recipes ........................................................................121

1. Chewy Breakfast Brownies........................................................121

2. Peach Banana Baked Oatmeal ..................................................122

3. Healthy Poppy seed Baked Oatmeal..........................................123

4. Healthy Berry Baked Oatmeal...................................................124

5. Apple Oatmeal Bars.................................................................124

6. Walnut Banana Bread .............................................................125

7. Cinnamon Zucchini Bread........................................................126

8. Italian Breakfast Bread...........................................................127

9. Coconut Zucchini Bread...........................................................128

10. Protein Banana Bread ...........................................................129

11. Easy Kale Muffins .................................................................130

12. Mouthwatering Shredded BBQ Roast.......................................131

13. Sour and Spicy Spareribs ......................................................132

14. Tender Pork Shoulder with Hot Peppers...................................133

15. Braised Sour Pork Filet..........................................................133

16. Pork with Anise and Cumin Stir-Fry ............................ 135

17. Baked Meatballs with Goat Cheese ............................ 136

18. Parisian Schnitzel ............................ 138

19. Kato Beef Stroganoff ............................ 139

20. Meatloaf with Gruyere ............................ 140

21. Roasted Filet Mignon in Foil ............................ 142

22. Stewed Beef with Green Beans ............................ 143

23. Garlic Herb Butter Roasted Radishes ............................ 144

24. Sausage-Stuffed Mushroom Caps ............................ 145

25. Cheesy Cauliflower Tots ............................ 145

26. Crispy Brussels sprouts ............................ 148

27. Zucchini Parmesan Chips ............................ 149

28. Roasted Garlic ............................ 150

30. Buffalo Cauliflower ............................ 153

31. Green Bean Casserole ............................ 154

32. Cilantro Lime Roasted Cauliflower ............................ 155

33. Dinner Rolls ............................ 156

34. Fiery Stuffed Peppers ............................ 157

35. Beef and veggies stir fry ............................ 158

36. Air Fried Chili Beef with Toasted Cashews ............................ 159

37.Beef Stir Fry W/ Red Onions & Peppers......................................160

38.Air Fryer Toast Oven Italian Beef................................................161

39.Healthy Quinoa Bowl with Grilled Steak & Veggies..................162

40.Pork Satay.....................................................................................163

41.Pork Burgers with Red Cabbage Salad ....................................164

42.Crispy Mustard Pork Tenderloin ...............................................165

43.Apple Pork Tenderloin ................................................................165

44.Espresso-Grilled Pork Tenderloin .............................................166

45.Garlic Lamb Chops with Thyme .................................................166

46.Lamb Meatloaf..............................................................................168

47.Lamb Chops and Mint Sauce......................................................169

48.Rosemary Roasted Lamb Cutlets ..............................................170


49.Seasoned Lamb............................................................................171

50.Herbed Lamb ...............................................................................172

51.Rack of Lamb ...............................................................................172

52.Lamb Sirloin Steak ......................................................................173

53.Beef Pork Meatballs ....................................................................174

54.Beef Noodle Casserole................................................................175

55.Saucy Beef Bake..........................................................................176

56.Beets and Arugula Salad ............................................................177

57.Beet Tomato and Goat Cheese Mix ...........................................178

58.Broccoli Salad ..............................................................................179

59.Brussels Sprouts and Tomatoes Mix.........................................180

60.Brussels Sprouts and Butter Sauce ..........................................180

61.Cheesy Brussels sprouts ............................................................181

62.Spicy Cabbage.............................................................................181

63.Sweet Baby Carrots Dish ............................................................182

64.Collard Greens Mix .................................................................183

65.Collard Greens and Turkey Wings.........................................184

66.Herbed Eggplant and Zucchini Mix.......................................185

67.Flavored Fennel .....................................................................185

68.Okra and Corn Salad..............................................................186

69.Air Fried Leeks.......................................................................187

70.Crispy Potatoes and Parsley..................................................188

71.Indian Turnips Salad .............................................................188

72.Simple Stuffed Tomatoes ......................................................189

73.Indian Potatoes......................................................................190

74.Broccoli and Tomatoes Air Fried Stew..................................191

75.Collard Greens and Bacon.....................................................191

76.Sesame Mustard Greens ........................................................192

77.Radish Hash ...........................................................................193

78.Cod Pie with Palmit ..............................................................193

79.Simple and Yummy Cod.........................................................194

80.Roasted Tilapia Fillet ...........................................................195

81. Cod 7-Mares ........................................................................196

82.Roasted Hake with Coconut Milk..........................................197

83.Air fryer Catfish....................................................................198

84.Squid to the Milanese............................................................199

85.Portugal Codfish with Cream ................................................199

86.Roasted Salmon with Provencal ...........................................200

87.Breaded Fish with Tartar Sauce ...........................................201

88.Milanese Fish Fillet ..............................................................202

89.Sole with White Wine ...........................................................202

90.Golden Fish with Shrimps ................................................203

91.Stroganoff Cod ................................................204

92.Cod Balls ................................................205

93.Lobster Bang Bang ................................................206

94.Honey Glazed Salmon ................................................206

95.Crispy Fish Fillet ................................................207

96.Garlic Butter Lobster Tails ................................................208

97.Pesto Fish ................................................209

98.Mozzarella Spinach Quiche ................................................209

99.Cheesy Zucchini Quiche ................................................210

100.Healthy Asparagus Quiche ................................................211

Conclusion ................................................213

# THE AIR FRYER RECIPES

**Table of Contents**

Introduction ..................................................................... 217

Recipes .......................................................................... 218

  1.Mini Veggie Quiche Cups ......................................... 218

  2.Lemon Blueberry Muffins ......................................... 220

  3.Baked Breakfast Donuts ........................................... 222

  4.Blueberry Almond Muffins ....................................... 223

  5.Feta Broccoli Frittata .............................................. 224

  6.Creamy Spinach Quiche .......................................... 226

  7.Turkey and Quinoa Stuffed Peppers ......................... 227

  8.Curried Chicken, Chickpeas and Raito Salad ............. 228

  9.Balsamic Vinaigrette on Roasted Chicken ................. 231

  10.Chicken Pasta Parmesan ....................................... 232

  11.Chicken and White Bean ........................................ 233

  12.Chicken Thighs with Butternut Squash .................... 235

  13.Cajun Rice & Chicken ............................................ 236

  14.Vegetable Lover's Chicken Soup ............................. 237

  15.Coconut Flour Cheesy Garlic Biscuits ..................... 239

  16.Radish Chips ........................................................ 240

  17.Flatbread ............................................................. 240

  18.Avocado Fries ...................................................... 241

  19.Pita-Style Chips .................................................... 242

  20.Roasted Eggplant .................................................. 242

  21.Parmesan-Herb Focaccia Bread .............................. 243

  22.Quick and Easy Home Fries ................................... 244

23. Jicama Fries ...................................................................245

24. Fried Green Tomatoes ..................................................246

25. Fried Pickles .................................................................246

26. Pork and Potatoes.........................................................247

27. Pork and Fruit Kebabs...................................................248

28. Steak and Vegetable Kebabs.......................................248

29. Spicy Grilled Steak........................................................249

30. Greek Vegetable Skillet ...............................................250

31. Light Herbed Meatballs.................................................250

32. Brown Rice and Beef-Stuffed Bell Peppers ...................251

33. Beef and Broccoli .........................................................252

34. Beef and Fruit Stir-Fry ...................................................252

35. Perfect Garlic Butter Steak ...........................................253

36. Crispy Pork Medallions .................................................254

37. Parmesan Meatballs .....................................................255

38. Tricolor Beef Skewers ....................................................256

39. Yogurt Beef Kebabs ......................................................257

40. Agave Beef Kebabs.......................................................258

41. Beef Skewers with Potato Salad ....................................259

42. Classic Souvlaki Kebobs................................................261

43. Harissa Dipped Beef Skewers ........................................262

44. Onion Pepper Beef Kebobs............................................263

45. Mayo Spiced Kebobs ....................................................264

46. Beef with Orzo Salad......................................................265

47. Beef Zucchini Shashliks...................................................266

48. Delicious Zucchini Mix ...................................................267

49. Swiss Chard and Sausage .............................................268

50. Swiss Chard Salad.........................................................269

51. Spanish Greens ..............................................................269

52. Flavored Air Fried Tomatoes .......................................................... 270

53. Italian Eggplant Stew ................................................................ 271

54. Rutabaga and Cherry Tomatoes Mix ................................................ 272

55. Garlic Tomatoes ..................................................................... 273

56. Tomato and Basil Tart ............................................................... 273

57. Zucchini Noodles Delight ............................................................ 275

58. Simple Tomatoes and Bell Pepper Sauce ........................................... 275

59. Salmon with Thyme & Mustard ..................................................... 276

60. Lemon Garlic Fish Fillet ............................................................. 277

61. Blackened Tilapia .................................................................... 278

62. Fish & Sweet Potato Chips ........................................................... 278

63. Brussels Sprout Chips ................................................................ 279

64. Shrimp Spring Rolls with Sweet Chili Sauce ....................................... 280

65. Coconut Shrimp and Apricot ........................................................ 281

66. Coconut Shrimp and Lime Juice .................................................... 283

67. Lemon Pepper Shrimp ............................................................... 284

68. Air Fryer Shrimp Bang ............................................................... 285

69. Crispy Nachos Prawns ............................................................... 286

70. Coconut Pumpkin Bars ............................................................... 286

71. Almond Peanut Butter Bars .......................................................... 287

72. Delicious Lemon Bars ................................................................ 288

73. Easy Egg Custard .................................................................... 289

74. Flavors Pumpkin Custard ............................................................ 290

75. Almond Butter Cookies .............................................................. 291

76. Tasty Pumpkin Cookies .............................................................. 292

77. Almond Pecan Cookies .............................................................. 293

78. Butter Cookies ...................................................................... 294

79. Tasty Brownie Cookies .............................................................. 295

80. Tasty Gingersnap Cookies .......................................................... 295

81.Simple Lemon Pie..................................................................296

82.Flavorful Coconut Cake ...........................................297

83.Easy Lemon Cheesecake.......................................................298

84.Lemon Butter Cake ....................................................299

85.Cream Cheese Butter Cake ...........................................300

86.Easy Ricotta Cake....................................................................300

87.Strawberry Muffins...................................................................301

88.Mini Brownie Muffins.............................................................302

89.Cinnamon Cheesecake Bars ........................................303

90.Strawberry Cobbler..............................................................304

91.Baked Zucchini Fries..............................................................305

92.Roasted Heirloom Tomato with Baked Feta ...................306

93.Garam Masala Beans.............................................................307

94.Crisp Potato Wedges .........................................................308

95.Crispy Onion Rings.................................................................309

96.Cheese Lasagna and Pumpkin Sauce ...........................309

97.Pasta Wraps...........................................................................311

98.Homemade Tater Tots...........................................................312

99.Mushroom, Onion, and Feta Frittata ...............................312

100.Roasted Bell Pepper Vegetable Salad ..........................314

Conclusion..............................................................................315

# Air Fryer Cookbook

## 100 Quick, Easy and Delicious Affordable Recipes for beginners

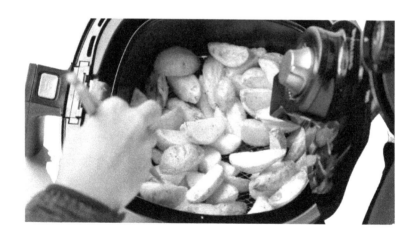

By Marisa Smith

## Introduction

Air fryers use dry air and less oil to cook your food. As per an estimation, 40 calories are found per teaspoon of oil (120 calories per tablespoon). The small amount of fat you add makes the results all too delicious and extra crispy to brown and caramelize. The amount you can see in the air fryer is basically nothing compared to the amount of oil in deep-fried foods, contributing to fewer calories than the normal fried food when saturated fat. The benefits of using an air freezer actually outweigh the risks. Besides that, the food turns out crispy and crunchy.

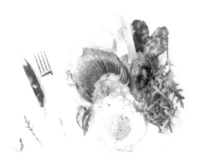

# Air Fryer Recipes

## 1.Squash Oat Muffins

Total time: 30 min

Prep time: 10 min

Cook time: 20 min

Yield: 12 servings

### Ingredients:

- Two eggs
- 1 tbsp. pumpkin pie spice
- 2 tsp. baking powder
- 1 cup oats
- 1 cup all-purpose flour
- 1 tsp. vanilla
- 1/3 cup olive oil
- 1/2 cup yogurt
- 1/2 cup maple syrup
- 1 cup butternut squash puree
- 1/2 tsp. sea salt

### Directions:

1. Strip 12 cups of a cupcake muffin tin with liners.

2. Wire rack insertion at rack position 6. Pick bake, set temperature to 390 f, 20-minute timer. To preheat the oven, press start.

3. Whisk together the milk, vanilla, oil, yogurt, maple syrup, and squash puree in a large bowl.

4. Mix together the rice, pumpkin pie spice, baking powder, oatmeal and salt in a shallow dish.

5. Apply the mixture of flour to the mixture and whisk to blend.

6. Scoop the batter and bake it for 20 minutes in a prepared muffin tin.

7. Enjoy and serve.

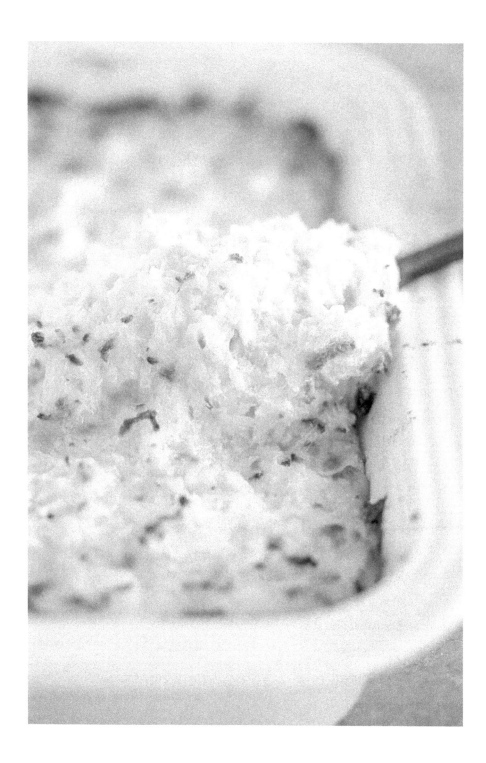

## 2.Hash brown Casserole

Total time: 1 hour 10 min

Prep time: 10 minutes

Cook time: 60 minutes

Yield: 10 servings

### Ingredients:

- 32 oz. frozen hash browns with onions and peppers
- 2 cups cheddar cheese, shredded
- 15 eggs, lightly beaten
- Five bacon slices, cooked and chopped
- Pepper
- Salt

### Directions:

1. Spray 9*13-inch casserole dish with cooking spray and set aside.
2. Insert wire rack in rack position 6. Select bake, set temperature 350 f, timer for 60 minutes. Press start to preheat the oven.
3. In a large mixing bowl, whisk eggs with pepper and salt. Add 1 cup cheese, bacon, and hash browns and mix well.
4. Pour egg mixture into the prepared casserole dish and sprinkle with remaining cheese.
5. Bake for 60 minutes or until the top is golden brown.
6. Slice and serve.

## 3.Mexican Breakfast Frittata

Prep time: 10 minutes

Cook time: 25 minutes

Yield: 6 servings

### Ingredients:

- 8 eggs, scrambled

- 1/2 cup cheddar cheese, grated
- 3 scallions, chopped
- 1/3 lb. tomatoes, sliced
- 1 green pepper, chopped
- 1/2 cup salsa
- 2 tsp. taco seasoning
- 1 tbsp. olive oil
- 1/2 lb. ground beef
- Pepper
- Salt

## Directions:

1. Spray a baking dish with cooking spray and set it aside.
2. Insert wire rack in rack position 6. Select bake, set temperature 375 f, timer for 25 minutes. Press start to preheat the oven.
3. Heat oil in a pan over medium heat. Add ground beef to a pan and cook until brown.
4. Add salsa, taco seasoning, scallions, and green pepper into the pan and stir well.
5. Transfer meat into the prepared baking dish. Arrange tomato slices on top of the meat mixture.
6. In a bowl, whisk eggs with cheese, pepper, and salt. Pour egg mixture over meat mixture and bake for 25 minutes.
7. Serve and enjoy.

## 4.Perfect Brunch Baked Eggs

Total time: 30 min

Prep time: 10 minutes

Cook time: 20 minutes

Servings: 4

## Ingredients:

- 4 eggs
- 1/2 cup parmesan cheese, grated
- 2 cups marinara sauce
- Pepper
- Salt

## Directions:

1. Spray with cooking spray on four shallow baking dishes and set aside.

2. Wire rack insertion at rack position 6. Pick bake, set temperature to 390 f, 20-minute timer. To preheat the oven, press start.

3. Divide the marinara sauce into four plates for baking.

4. Through each baking dish, split the egg. Sprinkle the eggs with cheese, pepper, and salt and bake for 20 minutes.

5. Enjoy and serve.

## 5. Green Chile Cheese Egg Casserole

Prep time: 10 minutes

Cook time: 40 minutes

Yield: 12 servings

## Ingredients:

- 12 eggs
- 8 oz. can green chilies, diced
- 6 tbsp. butter, melted
- 3 cups cheddar cheese, shredded
- 2 cups curd cottage cheese
- 1 tsp. baking powder
- 1/2 cup flour
- Pepper
- Salt

## Directions:

1.   Spray a 9*13-inch baking dish with cooking spray and set aside.

2.   Insert wire rack in rack position 6. Select bake, set temperature 350 f, timer for 40 minutes. Press start to preheat the oven.

3.   In a large mixing bowl, beat eggs until fluffy. Add baking powder, flour, pepper, and salt.

4.   Stir in green chilies, butter, cheddar cheese, and cottage cheese.

5.   Pour egg mixture into the prepared baking dish and bake for 40 minutes.

6.   Slice and serve.

## 6.Kale Zucchini Bake

Prep time: 10 minutes

Cook time: 30 minutes

Yield: 4 servings

### Ingredients:

- 1 onion, chopped
- 1 cup zucchini, shredded and squeezed out all liquid
- 1/2 tsp. dill
- 1/2 tsp. oregano
- Six eggs
- 1 cup cheddar cheese, shredded
- 1 cup kale, chopped
- 1/2 tsp. basil
- 1/2 tsp. baking powder
- 1/2 cup almond flour
- 1/2 cup milk
- 1/4 tsp. salt

### Directions:

1. With cooking oil, spray a 9*9-inch baking dish and put it aside.

2. Wire rack insertion at rack position 6. Pick bake, set temperature to 375 f, 35-minute timer. To preheat the oven, press start.

3. Whisk the eggs with the milk in a large mixing cup. Add the remaining ingredients, stirring until well mixed.

4. In the prepared baking dish, add in the egg mixture and bake for 35 minutes.

5. Slicing and cooking.

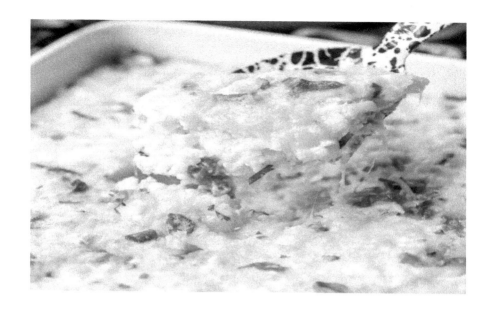

### 7.Cheesy Breakfast Casserole

Total time: 1 hour 10 min

Prep time: 10 min

Cook time: 60 min

Yield: 6 servings

**Ingredients:**

- 4 eggs
- 2 cups of milk
- 1 1/2 cup cheddar cheese, shredded
- Five bread slices, cut into cubes
- Pepper
- Salt

**Directions:**

1. Spray one 1/2-quart of baking dish and set aside with cooking spray.

2. Layer cubes of bread and alternately shredded cheese in a prepared baking dish.

3. Whisk the eggs with sugar, pepper and salt in a bowl and spill over the bread mixture. Put in the refrigerator overnight with a baking bowl.

4. Insert wire rack in place of rack 6. Pick bake, set temperature to 350 f, 60-minute timer. To preheat the oven, press start.

5. Take the baking dish out of the oven. For 60 minutes, roast.

6. Slicing and cooking.

## 8.Easy Hash Brown Breakfast Bake

Total time: 55 min

Prep time: 10 min

Cook time: 45 min

Yield: 8 servings

### Ingredients:

- 8 eggs
- 1 cup cheddar cheese, shredded
- 1 lb. bacon slices, cooked and crumbled
- Pepper
- 30 oz. frozen cubed hash brown potatoes, thawed
- 2 cups of milk
- Salt

### Directions:

1. Spray a 13*9-inch baking dish with cooking spray and set aside.
2. Insert wire rack in rack position 6. Select bake, set temperature 350 f, timer for 45 minutes. Press start to preheat the oven.
3. Add hash brown, bacon, and 1/2 cup cheese into the prepared baking dish.
4. In a bowl, whisk eggs with milk, pepper, and salt and pour over hash brown mixture. Sprinkle with remaining cheese and bake for 45 minutes.
5. Slice and serve.

## 9.Mexican Chiles Breakfast Bake

Total time: 50 min

Prep time: 10 min

Cook time: 40 min

Yield: 15 servings

## Ingredients:

- Six eggs
- 20 oz. hash brown potatoes, shredded
- 1/4 tsp. ground cumin
- 1/2 cup milk
- 2 cups Mexican cheese, shredded
- 1 lb. pork sausage, cooked and crumbled
- 1 cup chunky salsa
- 28 oz. can whole green chilies
- Pepper
- Salt

## Directions:

1. Spray a 13*9-inch baking dish with cooking spray and set aside.
2. Insert wire rack in rack position 6. Select bake, set temperature 350 f, timer for 40 minutes. Press start to preheat the oven.
3. Layer half potatoes, chilies, salsa, half sausage, and half cheese into the prepared baking dish. Cover with remaining sausage, potatoes, and cheese.
4. In a bowl, whisk eggs with milk, cumin, pepper, and salt and pour over potato mixture and bake for 40 minutes.
5. Serve and enjoy.

## 10.Delicious Amish Baked Oatmeal

Total time: 40 min

Prep time: 10 min

Cook time: 30 min

Yield: 8 servings

## Ingredients:

- Two eggs
- 3 cups rolled oats

- 1 tsp. cinnamon
- 1 1/2 tsp. vanilla
- 1 1/2 tsp. baking powder
- 1/4 cup butter, melted
- 1/2 cup maple syrup
- 1 1/2 cups milk
- 1/4 tsp. salt

## Directions:

1. Spray an 8*8-inch baking dish with cooking spray and set aside.
2. Insert wire rack in rack position 6. Select bake, set temperature 350 f, timer for 30 minutes. Press start to preheat the oven.
3. In a large bowl, whisk eggs with milk, cinnamon, vanilla, baking powder, butter, maple syrup, and salt. Add oats and mix well.
4. Pour mixture into the baking dish and bake for 30 minutes.
5. Slice and serve with warm milk and fruits.

## 11.Pork Sirloin Steak

Total time: 55 min

Prep time: 40 min

Cook time: 15 min

Yield: 2 servings

## Ingredients:

- 1/2 onion
- 1 teaspoon ginger powder
- 1 teaspoon garlic powder
- 1 teaspoon ground cinnamon
- 1/2 teaspoon ground cardamom
- 1/2 - 1 teaspoon cayenne
- 1 teaspoon salt

- 1-pound boneless pork sirloin steaks

## Directions:

1. Start by seasoning the steaks with pork loin. A generous amount of black pepper and salt, with a slight sprinkle of dried sage, is all you want to use. Don't be shy when it comes to seasoning. Before proceeding, making sure to season all sides of all the steaks properly.

2. On medium to high heat, melt a tablespoon of butter in a skillet. I want to wait until the cooking and bubbling of the butter begins. This means that the entire pan is heavy. This recipe for pork loin steak requires butter, not cooking spray or grease. Cooking steaks in butter adds so much flavor to them, and I notice that juicy steaks are created in this way.

3. It's time to add the steaks when the pan is heated, and the butter is melting and fried. You can cook 1 or 2 of them at a time. Just make sure you're not overfilling your plate. Leave it to cook until faint signs of browning begin to surface on the underside, then turn and cook on the other side. This is 4-5 minutes of cooking time on either side.

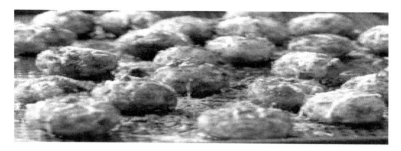

### 12.Chicken Meatballs with Cream Sauce and Cauliflower

Prep time: 40 min

Cook time: 15 min

Yield: 2 servings

**Ingredients:**

- 10 oz. Ground chicken
- 1 egg
- 2 oz. Grated parmesan cheese
- 1 teaspoon salt
- ½ teaspoon pepper
- 1 teaspoon dried basil
- 2 tablespoons sun-dried tomatoes in oil
- 1 tablespoon butter
- 1 lb. cauliflower
- 2 tablespoons butter for serving
- Cream sauce
- 1¼ cups coconut cream
- 1 tablespoon tomato paste
- 3 tablespoons finely chopped
- Fresh basil

**Directions:**

1. Combine the ground chicken ingredients and use a spoon to make 10 to 12 large balls (per pound). Following the manufacturer's instructions, ready the fryer. With a paper towel, gently coat the basket with elongated coconut oil and bake at 350 degrees for 10-13 minutes until lightly browned. Bring the oven back in and cook for another 4 to 5 minutes.

2. Place it on a plate after frying, then apply the cream and tomato paste. Let it cook over medium heat for 10 minutes.

3. With salt and pepper, season. Just before serving, add the fresh basil and cook the cauliflower for a few minutes in gently salted water. Serve alongside the chicken balls and cream sauce with a spoonful of sugar.

## 13.Shrimp Salad

Total time: 25 min

Prep time: 10 min

Cook time: 15 min

Yield: 2 servings

**Ingredients:**

- The salad
- 6 leaves lettuce
- 300 grams peeled shrimp
- 1 ½ tablespoon avocado oil
- ½ cup chopped celery
- 1 stalk chopped leek
- 4 tablespoons Greek yogurt
- 1 tablespoon coconut cream
- ½ teaspoon mint
- ½ teaspoon dried basil
- ¼ teaspoon chili powder
- 1 teaspoon lime juice

**Directions:**

1. Place the shrimp in the frying basket in one layer and air fried in the oven at 400 ° f for 10-14 minutes, depending on the size of the shrimp.

2. In a cup, mix together Greek yogurt, coconut milk, mint, dried basil, chili powder and lime juice.

3. Using the sliced celery and leek to place the fried shrimp in the dish. Combine the shrimp and vegetables before the dressing is covered.

4. Divide the lettuce and fill with the salad into separate portions.

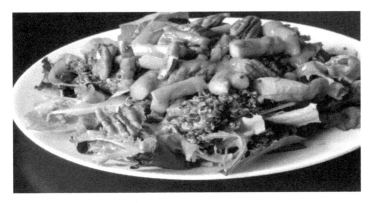

**14.Maple Asparagus Salad with Pecans**

Total time: 25 min

Prep time: 10 min

Cook time: 15 min

Yield: 4 servings

**Ingredients:**

- 10 medium asparagus spears
- ½ cup cherry tomatoes halved
- ½ cup chopped pecans
- ½ cup crumbled feta cheese
- 1-1/2 tablespoons coconut oil
- 1 tablespoon maple syrup

**Directions:**

1. Clean and cut the rough ends of the asparagus and spray coconut oil on the asparagus.

2. In an air fryer, place the asparagus in the oven. Cook at 360 degrees for 6 to 10 minutes to be crispy. In a cup, put the tomato halves, the diced pecans and the grated feta cheese.

3. In a shallow bowl, combine the coconut oil with the maple syrup and add the asparagus to the salad mix. Pour over the salad with the dressing combination.

4. To ensure the ingredients are evenly covered, combine the lettuce.

### 15. Creamed Kale

Total time: 25 min

Prep time: 10 min

Cook time: 15 min

Yield: 4 servings

**Ingredients:**

- 1 10 ounces package frozen kale, thawed
- 1/2 cup onions, chopped
- 2 teaspoons garlic powder
- 4 ounces cream cheese, diced
- 1 teaspoon ground black pepper
- 1 teaspoon salt
- 1/2 teaspoon ground cinnamon
- 1/4 cup shredded goat cheese

**Directions:**

1. Grease a 6-inch pan and set it aside. Mix the kale, onion, garlic, diced cream cheese, salt, pepper and cinnamon in a medium bowl.
2. Pour into a greased pan and place the fryer at 350 ° f for 10 minutes. Open and mix the kale to mix the goat cheese through the kale and sprinkle the goat over it.
3. Set the fryer to 400 ° f for 5 minutes or until the cheese melts and turns brown.

### 16. Baked Zucchini

Total time: 25 min

Prep time: 10 min

Cook time: 15 min

Yield: 4 servings

**Ingredients:**

- 2 medium-large zucchinis

- 1 teaspoon coconut oil
- 2 teaspoons butter
- 1 teaspoon stevia
- 1/2 teaspoon nutmeg

## Directions:

4. Rub the zucchinis with olive oil
5. Place the zucchinis in the air fryer. Cook for 40 minutes at 400 degrees.
6. Remove the zucchinis from the air fryer and allow them to cool.
7. Slice them open and load 1 teaspoon of butter and stevia and 1/4 teaspoon of nutmeg into each.
8. Cooking time may vary because every air fryer brand is different.

## 17. Roasted Broccoli Avocado Soup

Total time: 20 min

Prep time: 10 min

Cook time: 10 min

Yield: 4 servings

## Ingredients:

- 1 head broccoli
- 1 tablespoon garlic powder
- 2 cups chicken stock or vegetable stock
- 1 avocado peeled and cubed
- 1/2 lemon juiced
- 1 tablespoon coconut oil
- Sea salt to taste
- Fresh ground pepper to taste

## Directions:

9. Preheat the fryer to 390 degrees. Mix broccoli with garlic powder, salt and pepper and roast for 10 minutes. Carefully pour the broccoli with

the other ingredients into the blender at high speed and puree until it is smooth.

10. Add salt and pepper as desired, add water too thin to desired consistency if necessary and heat slightly over medium heat. Serve immediately.

## 18. Herbed Tuna

Total time: 20 min

Prep time: 10 min

Cook time: 10 min

Yield: 2 servings

### Ingredients:

- 8 oz. Sizzle fish tuna filets
- 1 teaspoon herbs
- 1/4 teaspoon sea salt
- 1/4 teaspoon black pepper
- 1/4 teaspoon smoked paprika
- 2 tablespoons coconut oil
- 1 tablespoon butter

### Directions:

1. Using a paper towel to dry fillets and run the surface carefully to ensure there are no bones.
2. Spray the fish with coconut oil and brush it on the two sides of the solution.
3. On both sides of the fish, combine the seasoning and scatter.
4. Cook an air fryer for 5-8 minutes at 390 degrees. Starting with 5 minutes, I suggest testing the fish and adding another minute to the time before it quickly crumbles with a fork.
5. In the oven, heat the seasoned butter for 30 seconds and spill it over the fish before eating.

## 19. Sirloin Steak

Total time: 20 min

Prep time: 10 min

Cook time: 10 min

Yield: 2 servings

**Ingredients:**

- 2 sirloin steaks
- Two tablespoons steak seasoning
- Coconut oil

**Directions:**

1. Using a paper towel to dry fillets and run the surface carefully to ensure there are no bones.
2. Spray the fish with coconut oil and brush it on the two sides of the solution.
3. On both sides of the fish, combine the seasoning and scatter.
4. Cook an air fryer for 5-8 minutes at 390 degrees. Starting with 5 minutes, I suggest testing the fish and adding another minute to the time before it quickly crumbles with a fork.
5. In the oven, heat the seasoned butter for 30 seconds and spill it over the fish before eating.

## 20. Whole Chicken

Total time: 1 hour 5 min

Prep time: 05 min

Cook time: 60 min

Yield: 4 servings

**Ingredients:**

- 1 (4-pound) whole chicken,
- 1 tablespoon coconut oil
- ¼ tablespoon kosher salt
- ½ teaspoon freshly ground black pepper
- ½ teaspoon garlic powder
- ½ teaspoon paprika (I prefer smoked paprika)
- ¼ teaspoon dried mint
- ¼ teaspoon dried oregano

- ¼ teaspoon dried thyme

## Directions:

1. Mix all of the spices into a paste with the oil and spread them all over the chicken.

2. Spray a basket of air fryers with an oil spray. Place the chicken in the basket face down and cook for 50 minutes at 360f.

3. Turn the chicken upside down and cook 10 minutes more.

4. Verify that there is an internal temperature of 165f in the breast chicken. Slice and serve.

## 21.Mini Sweet Pepper Poppers

Total time: 30 min

Prep time: 10 min

Cook time: 20 min

Yield: 4 (2 per servings)

## Ingredients:

- 8 mini sweet peppers
- 4 ounces of full-Fat: cream cheese, softened
- 4 slices of sugar-free bacon, cooked and crumbled
- 1/4 cup of shredded pepper jack cheese

## Directions:

1. Cut the pepper tops and slice on half lengthwise each. To cut seeds and membranes using a small knife.

2. Put together the cream cheese, bacon, and pepper jack in a shallow bowl.

3. In each sweet pepper, put 3 teaspoons of the mixture and press smoothly hard—place in basket fryer.

4. Set the temperature to 400° F, and set the timer for eight minutes.

5. Serve and enjoy!

## 22.Spicy Spinach Artichoke Dip

Total time: 30 min

Prep time: 10 min

Cook time: 20 min

Yield: (2 per servings)

**Ingredients:**

- 10 ounces of frozen spinach, drained and thawed
- 1 (14-ounce) can of artichoke hearts, drained and chopped
- 1/4 cup of chopped pickled jalapenos
- 8 ounces of full-Fat: cream cheese, softened
- 1/4 cup of full-Fat: mayonnaise
- 1/4 cup of full-Fat: sour cream
- 1/2 teaspoon of garlic powder
- ¼ cup of grated Parmesan cheese
- 1 cup of shredded pepper jack cheese

**Directions:**

1. In a 4-cup baking dish, combine the ingredients. In the Air Fryer, bring the basket in.
2. Fix the temperature for 10 minutes to 320° F and adjust the timer.
3. Start with an orange, then a bubble. Serve new and savor it!

## 23.Personal Mozzarella Pizza Crust

Total time: 30 min

Prep time: 10 min

Cook time: 20 min

Yield: (1per servings)

**Ingredients:**

- 1/2 cup of shredded whole-milk mozzarella cheese
- 2 tablespoons of blanched finely ground almond flour
- 1 tablespoon of full-Fat: cream cheese
- 1 large egg white

**Directions:**

1. In a medium microwave-safe bowl, place the mozzarella, almond flour, and cream cheese. Microwave that lasted 30 seconds. Stir until the dough ball forms smoothly. Add egg white and stir until the dough forms soft and round.

2. Press the crust of a 6 round pizza.

3. Cut a piece of parchment to fit your Air Fryer basket and place the crust on the parchment.

4. Set the temperature to 350° F and adjust the timer for 10 minutes.

5. Flip over the crust after 5 minutes and place any desired toppings at this time. Continue to cook until golden. Serve immediately.

## 24.Garlic Cheese Bread

Total time: 20 min

Prep time: 10 min

Cook time: 10 min

Yield: (2per servings)

### Ingredients:

- 1 cup of shredded mozzarella cheese
- 1/4 cup of grated Parmesan cheese
- 1 large egg
- 1/2 teaspoon of garlic powder

### Directions:

1. In a wide bowl, combine the ingredients. To suit your Air Fryer basket, cut a piece of parchment. Press the mixture in a circle onto the parchment, and put it in the Air Fryer basket.

2. Fix the temperature for 10 minutes to 350° F and adjust the timer.

3. Serve it warm and eat it!

## 25.Crustless Three-Meat Pizza

Total time: 20 min

Prep time: 10 min

Cook time: 10 min

Yield: (2per servings)

## Ingredients:

- 1/2 cup of shredded mozzarella cheese
- 7 slices of pepperoni
- 1/4 cup of cooked ground sausage
- 2 slices of sugar-free bacon, cooked and crumbled
- 1 tablespoon of grated Parmesan cheese
- 2 tablespoons of low-carb, sugar-free pizza sauce for dipping

## Directions:

1. Cover the bottom of the cake pan with mozzarella. Put the pepperoni, sausage, and bacon on top of the cheese and sprinkle with the Parmesan. Place the pan in the basket of the Air Fryer.

2. Change the temperature to 400° F and set a 5-minute timer.

3. Cut until the cheese is crispy and bubbling. Serve warm with a pizza sauce for dipping.

## 26.Smoky BBQ Roasted Almonds

Total time: 20 min

Prep time: 10 min

Cook time: 10 min

Yield:  (2per servings)

## Ingredients:

- 1 cup of raw almonds
- 2 teaspoons of coconut oil
- 1 teaspoon of chili powder
- 1/4 teaspoon of cumin
- 1/4 teaspoon of smoked paprika
- 1/4 teaspoon of onion powder

## Directions:

1. Put all the ingredients in a big bowl before the almonds are filled equally with oil and spices. Put the almonds in the Air Fryer box.

2. Fix the temperature for 6 minutes to 320° F and adjust the timer.

3. Halfway through the cooking process, remove the basket from the fryer. Enable it to totally cool off.

## 27.Beef Jerky

Total time: 20 min

Prep time: 10 min

Cook time: 10 min

Yield: (2per servings)

### Ingredients:

- 1-pound of flat iron beef, thinly sliced
- 1/4 cup of soy sauce
- 2 teaspoons of Worcestershire sauce
- 1/4 teaspoon of crushed red pepper flakes
- 1/4 teaspoon of garlic powder
- 1/4 teaspoon of onion powder

### Directions:

1. Place all the ingredients in a plastic bag or sealed container and marinate for 2 hours in the fridge.

2. On the Air Fryer rack, placed each jerky slice into a single sheet.

3. Fix the temperature to 160° F and for 4 hours, set the timer.

4. Up to 1 week of storage in airtight containers.

## 28.Pork Rind Nachos

Total time: 20 min

Prep time: 10 min

Cook time: 10 min

Yield: (2per servings)

### Ingredients:

- 1-ounce of pork rinds

- 4 ounces of shredded cooked chicken
- 1/2 cup of shredded Monterey jack cheese
- 1/4 cup of sliced pickled jalapeños
- 1/4 cup of guacamole
- 1/4 cup of full-Fat: sour cream

## Directions:

In a 6' round baking tray, put pork rinds. Fill with grilled chicken and cheese jack from Monterey. Place the Air Fryer in the basket with the plate.

Set the temperature to 370 degrees F and set the timer before the cheese is melted or for 5 minutes.

With jalapeños, guacamole, and sour cream, enjoy right now.

## 29.Ranch Roasted Almonds

Total time: 20 min

Prep time: 10 min

Cook time: 10 min

Yield:  (2per servings)

## Ingredients:

- 2 cups of raw almonds
- 2 tablespoons of unsalted butter, melted
- 1/2 (1-ounce) ranch dressing mix packet

## Directions:

1. To coat equally, stir the almonds in a large bowl of butter. Place almonds in the basket for Air Fryer Sprinkle ranch blend and sprinkle over almonds.

2. Fix the temperature for 6 minutes to 320° F and adjust the timer.

3. Shake the basket two or three times during training.

4. For at least 20 minutes, let it cool down. Almonds can become smooth during refrigeration to become crunchier. Place it in an air-tightened container for up to 3 days.

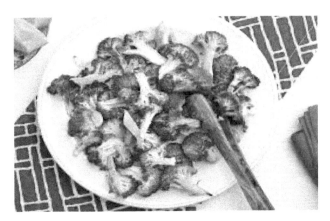

**30.Loaded Roasted Broccoli**

Total time: 20 min

Prep time: 10 min

Cook time: 10 min

Yield: (2per servings)

**Ingredients:**

- 3 cups of fresh broccoli florets
- 1 tablespoon of coconut oil
- 1/2 cup of shredded sharp Cheddar cheese
- 1/4 cup of full-Fat: sour cream
- 4slices of sugar-free bacon, cooked and crumbled
- 1 scallion, sliced

**Directions:**

1. Take the broccoli and drizzle it with coconut oil in the Air Fryer bowl.

2. Switch the temperature to 350 degrees F and set the timer for a further 10 minutes.

3. During exercise, toss a basket two or three times, or stop burning spots.

4. Remove from the fryer as the top begins to crisp the broccoli. Garnish with the melted cheese, sour cream, and crumbled bacon and scallion slices.

## 31. Scrumptious Leg of Lamb

Preparation time: 5 minutes

Cooking time: 1 hour

Servings: 4

### Ingredients:

- 1 1/4 kg leg of lamb
- 1 tablespoon olive oil
- A pinch of sea salt
- Pepper

### Directions:

1. Season the lamb's leg with salt and pepper and put it in the basket of the fryer.
2. Cook at 360 degrees for 20 minutes, turn the lamb's leg over and cook for a further 20 minutes.
3. Using roasted potatoes to serve.

## 32. Chinese Style Pork Chops

Preparation time: 15 minutes

Cooking time: 20 minutes

Servings: 4

### Ingredients:

- 450g Pork chops
- ¾ cup corn/potato starch
- 1 egg white
- ¼ tsp. Freshly ground black pepper
- ½ tsp. Kosher salt
- For the stir fry:
- 2 green onions, sliced
- 2 jalapeno peppers, seeds removed and sliced
- 2 tbsp. Peanut oil

- ¼ tsp. Freshly ground pepper and kosher salt to taste

## Directions:

1. Brush or spray with oil on the basket of your toast oven air fryer.

2. Next, mix the egg, salt and black pepper until it's frothy. Break up the pork chops and wipe the meat dry using a clean kitchen towel.

3. Toss the cutlets until evenly covered in the frothy egg mixture. For 30 minutes, cover and marinate.

4. Place the pork chops in a separate bowl and pour in the starch of corn/potato to ensure that each culet is dredged thoroughly. Shake off the extra corn/potato starch and place the prepared basket with the pork chops.

5. Set the air fryer toast oven to 360 degrees F and cook for 9 minutes, then shake the basket every 2-3 minutes, and if necessary, spray or brush the cutlets with more oil.

6. Increase the temperature to 400 degrees F and cook for another 6 minutes or until the chops are crisp.

7. Heat a wok or pan until incredibly hot over high heat. Apply all the ingredients for the stir fry and sauté for a minute.

8. Attach the pork chops you've fried and toss them with the stir fry.

9. Cook for another minute to guarantee that the stir-fry ingredients are uniformly mixed with the pork chops.

Enjoy!

### 33.Cinco De Mayo Pork Taquitos

Preparation time: 20 minutes

Cooking time: 15 minutes

Servings: 5

## Ingredients:

- 400g cooked and shredded pork tenderloin
- 10 flour tortillas2 ½ cups mozzarella, shredded
- 1 lemon, juiced
- Sour cream

- Salsa
- Cooking spray

## Directions:

1. Set your air fryer toast oven to 380 degrees f.

2. Squeeze the lemon juice over the shredded pork and mix well to combine.

3. Divide the tortillas into two and microwave, I batch at a time, covered with a slightly damp paper towel, so they don't become hard, for 15 seconds.

4. Divide the pork and cheese among the 10 tortillas.

5. Gently but tightly roll up all the tortillas.

6. Line your air fryer toast oven's pan with kitchen foil and arrange the tortillas on the pan.

7. Spray the tortillas with the cooking spray and cook for about 10 minutes, turning them over halfway through cook time.

8. Serve hot and enjoy!

## 34.Tangy Smoked Pork Chops with Raspberry Sauce

Preparation time: 15 minutes

Cooking time: 25 minutes

Servings: 4

## Ingredients:

- 4 medium-sized smoked pork chops
- 1 cup panko bread crumbs
- 2 eggs
- ¼ cup all-purpose flour
- ¼ cup milk
- 1 cup pecans, finely chopped
- 1/3 cup aged balsamic vinegar
- 2 tbsp. Raspberry jam, seedless
- 1 tbsp. Orange juice concentrate

- 2 tbsp. Brown sugar

## Directions:

1. Set your air fryer toast oven to 400 degrees f and spray/brush your air fryer toast oven's basket gently with oil.

2. Combine the milk and the eggs using a fork.

3. Mix the panko bread crumbs with the finely diced pecan in a separate bowl and place the flour in a third bowl.

4. Coat, one chop of pork at a time, of starch, brushing off the surplus.

5. Next, dunk the milk mixture and gently coat the crumb mixture on both sides. Gently pat to make the crumbs bind to the pork chops.

6. In the prepared basket, place the pork chops in one layer, spray lightly with cooking oil and cook for about 15 minutes, turning the chops halfway through the cooking time.

7. Combine all of the remaining ingredients in a pan over low-medium heat while the chops are frying. Carry to a boil until it thickens, then cook for 5-8 minutes.

8. Take out the chops and serve hot with the raspberry sauce.

9. Enjoy!

## 35.Air fryer toast oven bacon

Preparation time: 5 minutes

Cooking time: 15 minutes

Servings: 6

## Ingredients:

- 1/2 package (16 ounces) bacon

## Directions:

1. Preheat to 390° f with your air fryer toast cooker.

2. Arrange the bacon in the basket of the fryer in a single layer and cook for 8 minutes.

3. Flip the bacon over and cook for 7 more minutes or until crisp.

4. To drain excess grease, move it to a paper-lined tray.

5. Enjoy warm!

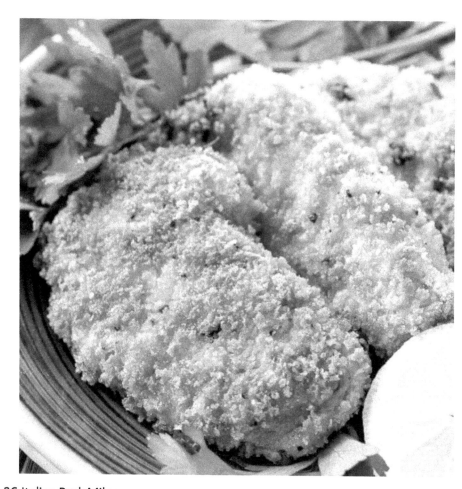

### 36.Italian Pork Milanese

Preparation time: 20 minutes

Cooking time: 10 minutes

Servings: 46

**Ingredients:**

- 6 pork chops, center-cut
- 2 eggs
- 2 tbsp. Water
- 1 cup panko bread crumbs seasoned with salt and black pepper
- ½ cup all-purpose flour

- 2 tbsp. Extra virgin olive oil
- Parmesan cheese, for serving (optional)
- For arugula salad:
- 1 bag fresh arugula
- 2 tbsp. Freshly squeezed lemon juice
- 1 tsp. Dijon mustard
- 1/8 cup extra virgin olive oil
- Freshly ground black pepper and sea salt to taste

## Directions:

1. To pound each chop of pork into 1/4 inch cutlets, use a mallet or rolling pin.

2. Season well with salt and pepper, then dip the flour into each cutlet. Shake the waste off.

3. In a small cup, whisk the eggs with water and dip the floured cutlets in the mixture, then roll them into the bread crumbs.

4. For all of the chops, do this and put it aside.

5. Set 380 degrees f for your air fryer toast oven.

6. Brush the breaded pork chops gently with olive and place the toast oven basket in one sheet on your air fryer. Cook for 3-5 minutes or until golden and crisp, then flip the chops and cook for another 3-5 minutes.

7. Meanwhile, in a large bowl, cook the salad by mixing the mustard, lemon juice, salt and pepper. With the vinaigrette, toss the arugula until finely covered.

8. Serve the arugula salad and top with crisp cutlets and parmesan cheese (optional). Enjoy!

## 37.Jamaican Jerk Pork Roast

Preparation time: 10 minutes

Cooking time: 1 hour 10 minutes

Servings: 10

**Ingredients:**

- 1800g pork shoulder
- 1 tbsp. Olive oil
- 1/4 cup Jamaican jerk spice blend
- 1/2 cup beef broth

**Directions:**

1. Set your air fryer to 400 degrees f and brown roast on both sides for 4 minutes on each side after rubbing the oil and seasoning.
2. Then decrease the temperature to 350 degrees f and bake for 1 hour, then remove from the fryer.
3.
4. Shred and serve.

## 38. Tasty and Moist Air Fryer Toast Oven Meatloaf

Preparation time: 20 minutes

Cooking time: 20 minutes

Servings: 4

**Ingredients:**

- 450 g lean minced meat
- 250 ml tomato sauce
- 1 small onion, finely chopped
- 1 tsp. Minced garlic
- 5 tbsp. Ketchup
- 1 tbsp. Worcestershire sauce
- 1/3 cup cornflakes crumbs
- 3 tsp. Brown sugar
- 1 ½ tsp. Freshly ground black pepper

- 1 ½ tsp. Sea salt
- 1 tsp. Dried basil
- ½ tsp. Freshly chopped parsley

**Directions:**

1. Combine the minced beef, corn flakes, chopped onion, garlic, basil, salt, pepper, and 3/4 of the tomato sauce in a large bowl. To blend and ensure that all the ingredients are mixed equally, use your hands.

2. Take your two shallow loaf pans and brush them loosely with vegetable oil. Divide the mixture of the meatloaf into two loaf pans.

3. Set the oven to 360 degrees f for your air fryer breakfast.

4. Combine the remainder of the tomato sauce, ketchup, Worcestershire sauce and brown sugar in a cup for the glaze. On the top and sides of the two loaves, rub this glaze blend.

5. Place the loaf pans, too, in the fryer. Cook and re-apply the glaze on the top and sides of the meatloaves for 10 minutes.

6. Cook for a further 10 minutes, twice in between, adding the glaze.

7. Sprinkle with the new parsley and cut the two loaf pans.

8. Before extracting the loaves from the loaf pans, let them stand for 3 minutes.

9. With mashed potatoes and a green salad, serve the perfectly moist and delicious meatloaf.

10. Enjoy!

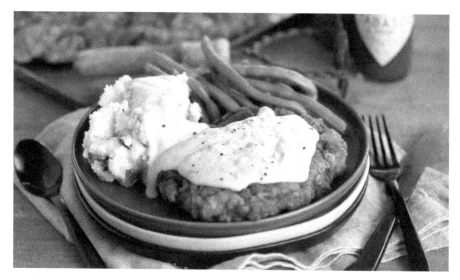

### 39.Classic Country Fried Steak

Preparation time: 15 minutes

Cooking time: 20 minutes

Servings: 2

**Ingredients:**

- 2 x 200g sirloin steaks
- 1 cup panko bread crumbs seasoned with kosher salt and freshly ground pepper
- 1 cup all-purpose flour
- 3 eggs, lightly beaten
- 1 tsp. Garlic powder
- 1 tsp. Onion powder
- For the sausage gravy:
- 150g ground sausage meat
- 2 cups milk
- 2 ½ tbsp. Flour
- 1 tsp. Freshly ground black pepper

**Directions:**

11. To pound the two steaks up to 1/2 - 1/4 inches thick, use a mallet or rolling pin.

12. In three separate shallow containers, placed the flour, egg and panko.

13. Dredge the steak in the flour first, then the egg and finally the bread crumbs then set them aside on a pan.

14. Brush the basket gently with oil from your air fryer toast oven, and then put the two breaded steaks on the basket.

15. Set the oven to 370 degrees f for the air fryer toast and cook the steak for 12 minutes, flipping once halfway through the cooking time.

16. Meanwhile, prepare the gravy by frying the sausage meat over medium-low heat in a pan until it browns uniformly. Drain the extra fat and reserve it in the pan for around a tablespoon or two.

17. Stir in the flour until well mixed, then, little by little, pour in the milk, stirring all the while.

18. For 3 minutes, season with freshly ground pepper and boil until the gravy is good and thick.

19. Using the sauce and some fluffy mashed potatoes to eat the steak. Yum!

## 40. Bourbon Infused Bacon Burger

Preparation time: 45 minutes

Cooking time: 30 minutes

Servings: 2

### Ingredients:

- 300g 80:20 lean ground beef
- 3 strips maple bacon, halved
- 1 small onion, minced
- 1 tbsp. Bourbon
- 2 tbsp. Bbq sauce
- 2 tbsp. Brown sugar
- 2 slices Monterey jack cheese
- Freshly ground black pepper, to taste
- Salt, to taste

- 2 burger rolls
- Sliced tomato for serving
- Torn lettuce, for serving
- For the sauce:
- 2 tbsp. Mayonnaise
- 2 tbsp. Bbq sauce
- ¼ tsp. Sweet paprika
- Freshly ground black pepper, to taste

## Directions:

1. Set your air fryer toast oven to 390 degrees F and pour around 1/2 cup of water into your air fryer toast oven's bottom drawer. This causes the smoking/burning grease to trickle away.

2. Mix the bourbon with the sugar. Arrange the strips of bacon in the basket of your air fryer toast oven and spray the tops with the sugar-bourbon mixture. Cook for 4 minutes, change the strips and brush with more sugar-bourbon mix and cook until brown and super crisp for 4 more minutes.

3. Meanwhile, the ground beef, chopped onion, salt, pepper and bbq sauce are mixed to create the burgers. To mix well, use your hands to make 2 burger patties.

4. If you like your burgers well cooked, set the air fryer toast oven at 370 degrees f and cook the burgers for 20 minutes, or 12-15 minutes if you like them medium-rare. Halfway into cooking time, flip the burgers.

5. Meanwhile, mix all the sauce ingredients in a bowl and stick them in the fridge to produce the sauce.

6. Cover each burger with a slice of Monterey Jack cheese for one minute of your cooking time. To keep the cheese from being blown away in the fryer, bind the cheese to the patty using a toothpick.

7. Cut each roll and spread the sauce on the sliced halves of the rolls to assemble the burger. Place one half of the burger and cover it with the bacon, tomatoes, lettuce and the other half of the roll. Enjoy!

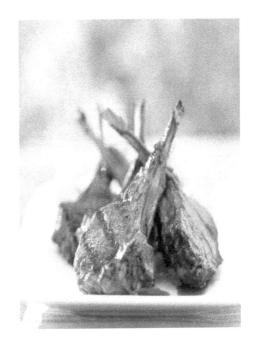

### 41.Glazed Lamb Chops

Preparation time: 10 minutes

Cooking time: 15 minutes

Servings: 4

**Ingredients:**

- 1 tablespoon dijon mustard
- ½ tablespoon fresh lime juice
- 1 teaspoon honey
- ½ teaspoon olive oil
- Salt and ground black pepper, as required
- 4 (4-ounce) lamb loin chops

**Directions:**

1. In a black pepper large bowl, mix the mustard, lemon juice, oil, honey, salt, and black pepper.
2. Add the chops and coat with the mixture generously.
3. Place the chops onto the greased "sheet pan."

4. Press the "power button" of the ninja food digital air fry oven and turn the dial to select the "air bake" mode.

5. Press the time button and again turn the dial to set the cooking time to 15 minutes.

6. Now push the temp button and rotate the dial to set the temperature at 390 degrees f.

7. Press the "start/pause" button to start.

8. When the unit beeps to show that it is preheated, open the lid.

9. Insert the "sheet pan" in the oven.

10. Flip the chops once halfway through.

11. Serve hot.

## 42.Buttered Leg of Lamb

Preparation time: 15 minutes

Cooking time: 1¼ hours

Servings: 8

**Ingredients:**

- 1 (2¼-pound) boneless leg of lamb
- 3 tablespoons butter, melted
- Salt and ground black pepper, as required
- 4 fresh rosemary sprigs

**Directions:**

1. Rub with butter on the leg of the lamb and sprinkle with salt and black pepper.

2. Wrap a leg of lamb with sprigs of rosemary.

3. "Press the ninja foodie digital air fry oven's "power button" and turn the dial to select the mode for "air fry.

4. To set the cooking time to 75 minutes, press the time button and change the dial once again.

5. Now press the temp button to set the temperature at 300 degrees f and rotate the dial.

6. To start, press the 'start/pause' button.

7. "Open the "air fry basket" lid and grease when the machine beeps to indicate that it is preheated.

8. Arrange the leg of lamb into an "air fry basket" and insert it in the oven.

9. Remove from the oven and put the lamb's leg on a cutting board before slicing for about 10 minutes.

10. Split into bits of the appropriate size and serve.

## 43.Glazed Lamb Meatballs

Preparation time: 20 minutes

Cooking time: 30 minutes

Servings: 8

## Ingredients:

- For meatballs:
- ½ cup Ritz crackers, crushed
- Salt and ground black pepper, as required
- 1 (5-ounce) can evaporate milk
- 2 large eggs, beaten lightly
- 1 tablespoon dried onion, minced
- 1 teaspoon maple syrup
- 2 pounds lean ground lamb
- 2/3 cup quick-cooking oats
- For sauce:
- 1/3 cup sugar
- 1/3 cup orange marmalade
- 1-2 tablespoons sriracha
- 1/3 cup maple syrup
- 1 tablespoon Worcestershire sauce
- 2 tablespoons cornstarch

- 2 tablespoons soy sauce

## Directions:

1. For meatballs: Put all the ingredients in a large bowl and mix until well mixed.

2. From the mixture, produce 11/2-inch balls.

3. Add half of the meatballs in a single layer to the greased "sheet pan."

4. "Press the ninja foodie digital air fry oven's "power button" and turn the dial to select the mode for "air fry.

5. To set the cooking time to 15 minutes, click the time button and change the dial once again.

6. Now press the temp button to set the temperature at 380 degrees f and rotate the dial.

7. To start, press the 'start/pause' button.

8. Open the lid when the device beeps to demonstrate that it is preheated.

9. Place the' sheet pan' in the oven.

10. Halfway through, turn the meatballs once.

11. Remove the meatballs from the oven and transfer them to a dish.

12. Repeat with the meatballs that remain.

13. Meanwhile, for sauce, put all the ingredients in a small pan: over medium heat and cook until thickened, stirring constantly.

14. Serve the meatballs with sauce on top.

## 44.Oregano Lamb Chops

Preparation time: 10 minutes

Cooking time: 30 minutes

Servings: 4

## Ingredients:

- 4 lamb chops
- 1 garlic clove, peeled
- 1 tbsp. plus

- 2 tsp. olive oil
- ½ tbsp. oregano
- ½ tbsp. thyme
- Salt and black pepper to taste

**Directions:**

1. Preheat the fryer to 390 f for air. Coat the clove of garlic with 1 tsp. Place the olive oil in the air fryer for 10 minutes. Meanwhile, with the remaining olive oil, combine the herbs and seasonings.

2. Squeeze the hot roasted garlic clove into the herb mixture using a towel or a mitten, and stir to blend. Cover the lamb chops well with the mixture and put them in the oven for frying. For 8 to 12 minutes, cook. Serve it warm.

### 45.Lamb Steaks with Fresh Mint and Potatoes

Preparation time: 10 minutes

Cooking time: 25 minutes

Servings: 2

**Ingredients:**

- 2 lamb steaks
- 2 tbsp. Olive oil
- 2 garlic cloves, crushed
- Salt and pepper, to taste
- A handful of fresh thyme, chopped
- 4 red potatoes, cubed

**Directions:**

1. Using oil, garlic, salt, and black pepper to rub the steaks. In the fryer, put the thyme and place the steaks on top. Oil the chunks of the potato and sprinkle them with salt and pepper. Arrange the potatoes next to the steaks and cook for 14 minutes at 360 f, turning once halfway through the cooking process.

### 46.Lamb Kofta

Preparation time: 6 minutes

Cooking time: 12 minutes

Servings: 4

## Ingredients:

- 1 pound ground lamb
- 1 tsp. cumin
- 2 tbsp. mint, chopped
- 1 tsp. garlic powder
- 1 tsp. onion powder
- 1 tbsp. ras el hanout
- ½ tsp. ground coriander
- 4 bamboo skewers
- Salt and black pepper to taste

## Directions:

2. Lamb, cumin, garlic powder, mint, onion powder, ras el hanout, cilantro, salt and pepper are combined in a cup. Place on skewers and mold into sausage shapes. Marinate it in the fridge for 15 minutes.

3. Preheat to 380 f with your air fryer. Spray a basket of air fryers with cooking spray. Arrange the skewers in the basket of an air fryer. Cook for 8 minutes, turning once halfway through. Serve with dip with yogurt.

## 47.Crunchy Cashew Lamb Rack

Preparation time: 10 minutes

Cooking time: 30 minutes

Servings: 4

## Ingredients:

- 3 oz. chopped cashews
- 1 tbsp. chopped rosemary
- 1 ½ lb. rack of lamb
- 1 garlic clove, minced

- 1 tbsp. breadcrumbs

- 1 egg, beaten

- 1 tbsp. olive oil

- Salt and pepper to taste

## Directions:

1. Heat the air-freezer to 210 f. Combine the garlic with the olive oil and spray this mixture over the lamb. In a dish, blend the rosemary, cashews, and crumbs. Brush the lambs with the egg, then cover them with the cashew mixture. Place the lamb in the basket of an air fryer and cook for 25 minutes. Increase the heat to 390 f, and cook for an additional 5 minutes. Cover with foil and leave to rest before serving for a few minutes.

## 48.Oregano & Thyme Lamb Chops

Preparation time: 10 minutes

Cooking time: 30 minutes

Servings: 4

## Ingredients:

- 4 lamb chops

- 1 garlic clove, peeled

- 1 tbsp. plus

- 2 tsp. olive oil

- ½ tbsp. oregano

- ½ tbsp. thyme

- ½ tsp. salt

- ¼ tsp. black pepper

## Directions:

2. Preheat the fryer to 390 f for air. Coat the clove of garlic with 1 tsp. Olive oil and put for 10 minutes in the air fryer. With the remaining olive oil, combine the herbs and seasonings.

3. Squeeze the hot roasted garlic clove into the herb mixture using a towel or a mitten, and stir to blend. Thoroughly coat the lamb chops with the mixture, and put in the air fryer. 12 minutes to cook.

## 49.Lamb Meatballs

Preparation time: 10 minutes

Cooking time: 40 minutes

Servings: 12

### Ingredients:

- 1 ½ lb ground lamb
- ½ cup minced onion
- 2 tbsp. chopped mint leaves
- 3 garlic cloves, minced
- 2 tsp. paprika
- 2 tsp. coriander seeds
- ½ tsp. cayenne pepper
- 1 tsp. salt
- 1 tbsp. chopped parsley
- 2 tsp. cumin
- ½ tsp. ground ginger

### Directions:

20. Soak 24 skewers in water until ready to use. Preheat the air fryer to 330 f. Combine all ingredients in a large bowl. Mix well with your hands until the herbs and spices are evenly distributed, and the mixture is well combined. Shape the lamb mixture into 12 sausage shapes around 2 skewers. Cook for 12 to 15 minutes, or until it reaches the preferred doneness. Served with tzatziki sauce and enjoy.

## 50.Thyme Lamb Chops with Asparagus

Preparation time: 10 minutes

Cooking time: 20 minutes

Servings: 4

**Ingredients:**

- 1 pound lamb chops
- 2tspolive oil
- 1½ tsp. chopped fresh thyme
- 1 garlic clove, minced
- Salt and black pepper to taste
- 4 asparagus spears, trimmed

**Directions:**

1. Preheat to 400 f with your air fryer. Spray a basket of air fryers with cooking spray.
2. Drizzle some olive oil with the asparagus, sprinkle with salt, and set aside with salt and black pepper, season the lamb. Brush and move the remaining olive oil to the cooking basket. Slide the basket out, transform the chops and add the asparagus. Cook for 10 minutes. For another 5 minutes, cook. Serve with thyme sprinkles.

### 51.Cornflakes French toast

Total time: 20 min

Prep time: 10 min

Cook time: 10 min

Yield: 2 servings

**Ingredients:**

- Bread slices (brown or white)
- 1 egg white for every 2 slices
- 1 tsp. of sugar for every 2 slices
- Crushed cornflakes

**Directions:**

1. Place two slices together, then trim them along the diagonal. In a bowl, whisk together the egg whites, then add a little sugar.
2. Immerse the bread triangles in this mixture and coat them with the crushed corn blossoms.

3. Preheat the Air Fryer at 180o C for 4 minutes. Place the triangles of coated bread in and close the box for frying. Let them cook for at least a further 20 minutes at the same temperature.

4. To get an even chef, turn the triangles over. Serve the slices of chocolate syrup.

## 52.Mint Galette

Total time: 10 min

Prep time: 5 min

Cook time: 5 min

Yield: 2 servings

### Ingredients:

- 2 cups of mint leaves (Sliced fine)
- 2 medium potatoes boiled and mashed
- 1 ½ cup of coarsely crushed peanuts
- 3 tsp. of ginger finely chopped
- 1-2 tbsp. of fresh coriander leaves
- 2 or 3 green chilies finely chopped
- 1 ½ tbsp. of lemon juice
- Salt and pepper to the taste

### Directions:

1. Mix the sliced mint leaves with the remaining ingredients in a clean dish. Shape this mixture into galettes that are flat and round.

2. Wet the galettes softly with sweat. Cover each peanut with each smashed galette.

3. Preheat the Air Fryer, at 160° Fahrenheit, for 5 minutes. Place the galettes in the frying bowl and let them steam at about the same temperature for another 25 minutes.

4. In order to get a cook that is even, keep turning them over. Using chutney, basil, or ketchup to serve.

## 53.Cottage Cheese Sticks

Total time: 10 min

Prep time: 5 min

Cook time: 5 min

Yield: 2 servings

## Ingredients:

- 2 cups of cottage cheese
- 1 big lemon-juiced
- 1 tbsp. of ginger-garlic paste

For seasoning, use salt and red chili powder in small amounts

- ½ tsp. of carom
- One or two papadums
- 4 or 5 tbsp. of cornflour
- 1 cup of water

## Directions:

1. Take the cheese and cut it into pieces that are long. Currently, a combination of lemon juice, red chili powder, spices, ginger garlic paste, and caramel is used as a marinade.

2. Marinate the slices of cottage cheese in the mixture for a bit, then wrap them in dry cornflour for about 20 minutes to set aside.

3. Take the papadum and cook it in a saucepan. Crush them until they are cooked into very tiny pieces. Take another bottle now and pour about 100 ml of water in it.

4. Loosen 2 tablespoons of cornflour in the water. Dip the cottage cheese pieces in this cornflour solution and roll them on to the bits of crushed papadum so that the papadum attaches to the cottage cheese.

5. Preheat the Air Fryer for 10 minutes at about 290 Fahrenheit. Then open the basket for the fryer and put the cottage cheese bits inside it. Cover the bowl well. Enable the fryer to sit at 160 ° for another 20 minutes.

6. Open the basket halfway through, and put a little of the cottage cheese around to allow for standard cooking. Until they're cooked,

you can eat them with either ketchup or mint chutney. Serve and chutney with mint.

## 54. Palak Galette

Total time: 20 min

Prep time: 10 min

Cook time: 10 min

Yield: 2 servings

### Ingredients:

- 2 tbsp. of garam masala
- 2 cups of Palak leaves
- 1 ½ cup of coarsely crushed peanuts
- 3 tsp. of ginger finely chopped
- 1-2 tbsp. of fresh coriander leaves
- 2 or 3 green chilies finely chopped
- 1 ½ tbsp. of lemon juice
- Salt and pepper to the taste

### Directions:

1. Blend into a clean container with the ingredients. Shape this mixture into galettes that are smooth and round. Wet the galettes softly with sweat. Coat up each galette with smashed peanuts.

2. Preheat the Air Fryer, at 160° Fahrenheit, for 5 minutes. Place the galettes in the basket and let them cook for another 25 minutes at the same temperature. Go turn them over to cook them. Using ketchup or mint chutney to serve.

## 55. Spinach Pie

Total time: 10 min

Prep time: 5 min

Cook time: 5 min

Yield: 2 servings

### Ingredients:

- 7 ounces of flour
- 2 tablespoons of butter
- 7ounces of spinach
- 1 tablespoon of olive oil
- 2 eggs
- 2 tablespoons of milk
- 3 ounces of cottage cheese
- Salt and black pepper to the taste
- 1 yellow onion, chopped

**Directions:**

1. In your food processor, mix flour and butter, 1 egg, milk, salt and pepper, combine properly, switch to a cup, knead, cover, and leave for 10 minutes.

2. Heat the pan with the oil over medium heat, add the spinach and onion, stir and simmer for 2 minutes.

3. Attach salt, pepper, cottage cheese, and leftover egg, stir well and heat up.

4. Divide the dough into 4 pieces, roll each piece, place it on a ramekin's rim, add the spinach filling over the dough, place the ramekins in your Air Fryer's basket, and cook at 360° F for 15 minutes.

5. Serve it sweet.

## 56.Balsamic Artichokes

Total time: 10 min

Prep time: 5 min

Cook time: 5 min

Yield: 7 servings

**Ingredients:**

- 4 big artichokes, trimmed
- Salt and black pepper to the taste
- 2 tablespoons of lemon juice

- ¼ cup of extra virgin olive oil
- 2 teaspoons of balsamic vinegar
- 1 teaspoon of oregano, dried
- 2 garlic cloves, minced

**Directions:**

1. Season the salt and pepper with the artichokes, rub them with half the oil and half the lemon juice, put them in your Air Fryer and cook at 360 ° F for 7 minutes.
2. Meanwhile, in a cup, combine the remaining lemon juice, vinegar, remaining oil, salt, pepper, garlic, and oregano and mix well.
3. Arrange the artichokes on a tray, coat them with a balsamic vinaigrette, and eat.

## 57.Cheesy Artichokes

Total time: 15 min

Prep time: 5 min

Cook time: 5 min

Yield: 7 servings

**Ingredients:**

- 14 ounces of canned artichoke hearts
- 8 ounces of cream cheese
- 16 ounces of parmesan cheese, grated
- 10 ounces of spinach
- ½ cup of chicken stock
- 8 ounces of mozzarella, shredded
- ½ cup of sour cream
- 3 garlic cloves, minced
- ½ cup of mayonnaise
- 1 teaspoon of onion powder

**Directions:**

1. In a saucepan appropriate for your Air Fryer, blend artichokes with stock, garlic, spinach, cream cheese, sour cream, onion powder and mayo, put in the Air Fryer, and cook for 6 minutes at 350 °F.
2. Apply the mozzarella and parmesan and then stir well and eat.

## 58.Artichokes and Special Sauce

Total time: 15 min

Prep time: 5 min

Cook time: 5 min

Yield: 2 servings

### Ingredients:

- 2 artichokes, trimmed
- A drizzle of olive oil
- 2 garlic cloves, minced
- 1 tablespoon of lemon juice

### For the sauce:

- ¼ cup of coconut oil
- ¼ cup of extra virgin olive oil
- 3 anchovy fillets
- 3 garlic cloves

### Directions:

1. Mix the artichokes with the oil, 2 cloves of garlic and lemon juice in a cup, toss well, move to your Air Fryer, and cook for 6 minutes at 350 ° F and split between plates.
2. Mix coconut oil with anchovy, 3 garlic cloves, and olive oil in your food processor, blend very well, drizzle with artichokes and eat.

## 59.Beet Salad and Parsley Dressing

Total time: 25 min

Prep time: 10 min

Cook time: 25 min

Yield: 4 servings

**Ingredients:**

- 4 beets
- 2 tablespoons of balsamic vinegar
- A bunch of parsley, chopped
- Salt and black pepper to the taste
- 1 tablespoon of extra-virgin olive oil
- 1 garlic clove, chopped
- 2 tablespoons of capers

**Directions:**

1. Place the beets and cook at 360 ° F for 14 minutes in your Air Fryer.
2. Meanwhile, in a dish, mix the parsley, garlic, salt, pepper, olive oil, and capers, and whisk very well.
3. Move the beets to a cutting board, cool them down, slice them, and place them in a salad bowl.
4. All over the parsley dressing, apply vinegar and drizzle and eat.

## 60.Beets and Blue Cheese Salad

Total time: 25 min

Prep time: 10 min

Cook time: 25 min

Yield: 6 servings

**Ingredients:**

- 6 beets, peeled and quartered
- Salt and black pepper to the taste
- ¼ cup of blue cheese, crumbled
- 1 tablespoon of olive oil

**Directions:**

1. In the Air Fryer, place the beets, cook them at 350 ° F for 14 minutes and then move them to a dish.

2. Apply the blue cheese, salt, pepper, and oil to the mixture, and then toss and eat.

## 61.Shrimp Pancakes

Preparation Time: 5 Minutes

Cooking Time: 15 Minutes

Servings: 10-12

### Ingredients:

- 1 cup all-purpose flour
- 1 glass of water
- 3 beaten eggs
- 1 tablet chicken broth

### Directions:

1. Boil the water and dissolve the chicken broth, let it cool and place the beaten eggs and the wheat flour, stir well until everything dissolves and a smooth mass fry the tablespoons and a little oil in the Tefal pan and keep the part in a baking dish.

2. Make the prawns taste and leave with a little sauce.

3. Top with pancakes and shrimp sauce and sprinkle with grated cheese. Do this until the last layers of grated cheese are ready.

4. Bake in the air fryer at 3600F for 15 minutes. Serve with white rice and salad.

## 62.Shrimps with Palmito

Preparation Time: 10 Minutes

Cooking Time: 30 Minutes

Servings: 4-8

### Ingredients:

### White Sauce:

- 1 cup grated Parmesan cheese
- 1 tbsp. butter
- 4 ½ lb shrimp

- ½ cup of olive oil
- Very minced garlic Striped onion
- 1 can of sour cream
- 1 can of sliced palm heart Grated Parmesan

## Sauce:

- 1 onion, sliced
- Margarine and butter
- 2 cups milk
- 2 tbsp. of flour
- Salt to taste
- cheese for sprinkling

## Preparation of the white sauce:

1. With the margarine and butter, lightly brown the onion.

2. In a blender, place the milk and wheat flour.

3. Add the onion which has been stewed.

4. Beat it all really well.

5. Bring this mixture to the fire and cook until a dense cream appears. Add the Parmesan cheese and butter and extract the white sauce from the heat. Reserve. Reserve.

6. Sauté the snails with garlic and onion in olive oil.

7. To the white sauce, add the sautéed shrimp and eventually add the palm kernel and milk, mixing it all very well.

8. Sprinkle plenty of Parmesan cheese on top, set in a greased refractory form.
9. Bake for 1520 minutes in the air-fryer at 3600F.

## 63.Gratinated Pawns with Cheese
Preparation Time: 10 Minutes

Cooking Time: 20 Minutes

Servings: 4

## Ingredients:

- 2 ¼ lbs. clean, chopped prawns
- 1 tbsp. of fondor
- 1 tbsp. of oil
- 1 tbsp. butter
- 1 grated onion
- 5 tomatoes, beaten in a blender
- 1 tablet of crumbled shrimp broth
- 1 glass of light cream cheese
- 1 tbsp. of breadcrumbs
- 1 tbsp. Parmesan cheese

**Directions:**

1. Use one such fondor to season the prawns and reserve for 1 hour.

2. In the oil and butter combination, cook them.

3. Position them and set them aside in a refractory container.

4. Brown, the onion in the fat of the shrimp, add the tomatoes, a tablet of the shrimp broth and a cup of boiling water.

5. Bring to a boil, until just a touch, in a covered skillet.

6. Add the curd, then stir until it freezes.

7. Pour over the prawns and sprinkle the mixed breadcrumbs with the grated rib.

8. Parmesan cheese and placed it in a 400oF air fryer for 20 minutes or until golden brown.

### 64.Air fryer Crab

Preparation Time: 5 Minutes

Cooking Time: 10 Minutes

Servings: 20

**Ingredients:**

- 1 pound of crab meat 20 crab cones
- 2 onions

- 2 tomatoes
- 3 garlic cloves
- 1 bell pepper
- ½ glass of white vinegar
- 1 head of black pepper
- 1 head of cumin
- 1 small salt
- Olive oil to taste

## Directions:

1. Place the onion that has been sliced until golden. Then, with 1⁄2 glass of vinegar, add the remaining spices (pepper, cumin, minced garlic).

2. Put in the green smell, the crushed tomatoes, and the cut pepper. Add the olive oil to taste when the seasoning is well done (at least 3 tablespoons).

3. Then add the meat to the crab and cook for 5 minutes.

4. Fill the crab cones, drizzle with grated Parmesan cheese and bake for 5 minutes in an air fryer at 3200 to melt the cheese.

## 65.Crab Balls

Preparation Time: 10 Minutes

Cooking Time: 20 Minutes

Servings: 2-4

## Ingredients:

- 1 lb of crab Salt to taste Olive oil
- 2 cloves garlic, minced
- 1 chopped onion
- 3 tbsp. of wheat flour
- 1 tbsp. of parsley
- 1 fish seasoning
- 2 lemons
- 1 cup milk

### Tarnish:

1. Wash the crab in the juice of 1 lemon.

2. Season with the juice of the other lemon, along with the salt and the prepared fish seasoning.

3. In a frying pan, sauté the onion and garlic with the sweet oil.

4. Mix the crab meat with the stir fry. 5. Let cook in this mixture for another 5 minutes.

6. Add the parsley.

7. Dissolve the flour in the milk and add it to the crab.

8. Stir constantly, until this mixture begins to come out of the pan.

9. Let cool, shape the meatballs, go through the beaten egg and breadcrumbs.

10. 1 beaten egg Bread crumbs Oil for frying

11. Fry in the air fryer at 4000F for 25 minutes.

### 66.Crab Empanada

Preparation Time: 15 Minutes

Cooking Time: 30 Minutes

Servings: 4-8

### Ingredients:

- 1 small onion
- 1 tomato
- 1 small green pepper
- 1 lb of crab meat Seasoning ready for fish
- 1 tbsp. of oil Pastry dough

### Directions:

1. In oil, sauté the chopped onion, tomato, and pepper.

2. Add the sauce and crab meat.

3. Cook, without stirring, until very dry so that it does not stick to the bottom of the pan.

4. Fill the cakes with the crab meat that has been prepared.

5. Fry it in an air fryer for 25 minutes at 4000F.

## 67.Crab Meat on Cabbage

Preparation Time: 10 Minutes

Cooking Time: 15 Minutes

Servings: 2-4

### Ingredients:

- 1 pound shredded crab meat
- 1 pound cooked and minced dogfish
- 2 cups of cooked rice
- 1 small green cabbage
- Parsley and coriander
- Chile
- 2 tbsp. of palm oil

### Directions:

1. In a little water, season and cook the dogfish.

2. Crush the broth that has been created when it is smooth and drink it. Add the crab meat, which should have been thawed already. Add the tomato sauce, palm oil, pepper and cooked rice.

3. In warm water, dissolve the starch and pour it into the mixture. Sharpen the mixture, taste the salt and brush on top with the chopped parsley and coriander.

4. Cook 6 whole leaves of cabbage separately, until al dente, in salted water.

5. Place the open leaves and crab cream with 2 tbsp. of cornstarch in a baking dish. Tomato sauce Bread crumbs Garlic fish inside.

7. Sprinkle with breadcrumbs and bake for 5 minutes in an air fryer at 3200F to brown.

## 68.Gratinated Cod

Preparation Time: 15 Minutes

Cooking Time: 45 Minutes

Servings: 4-8

## Ingredients:

- 2 ¼ lb cod
- 1 red bell pepper
- 1 green bell pepper
- 1 onion
- 3 ripe tomatoes
- 2 cloves of garlic
- 1 cup black olives
- Oregano to taste

## Cream:

- 1 cup catupiry cheese
- 1 can of cream
- ½ cup coconut milk

## Mashed potatoes:

1. First, prepare the mashed potatoes, squeeze the potatoes and, with the potatoes still very sweet, add the butter and cream, mix well and add salt to taste.

2. On a high ovenproof plate, put this puree. Then arrange yourself like a pie crust. Make the stir fry with the already desalted cod (soak the day before and change the water at least 5 times).

3. Bring to a boil briefly, in boiling water, for 5 minutes.

4. Crush the cod into chips, then.

5. In a frying pan, put ample oil and cook the onion and garlic. Then add 2 1/4 lb of boiled and squeezed potatoes 2 butter spoons 1/2 cup of milk Salt to taste Sour cream and bell peppers and simmer for about 10 minutes.

6. Then add the cod and olives and let it simmer for 10 further minutes.

7. Without letting so much of it dry out. And, to taste, apply oregano. You don't usually have to add salt since the cod already contains plenty of it.

8. If you need to bring in a bit, however.

9. Play over mashed potatoes with this braised cod. Cream:: Cream

10. In a blender, beat all the ingredients and pour over the cod.

11. For 30 minutes or until it is orange, take it to the previously heated air fryer at 6000F.

12. Serve with a leafy salad and white rice.

## 69.Gratinated Cod with Vegetables

Preparation Time: 10 Minutes

Cooking Time: 30 Minutes

Servings: 2-4

### Ingredients:

- 2 ¼ lb cod 1 pound of potato 1 pound carrot
- 2 large onions
- 2 red tomatoes
- 1 bell pepper
- 1 tbsp. of tomato paste
- Coconut milk
- Garlic, salt, coriander and olive oil to taste.
- Olives

### Sauce:

1. For 24 hours, soak the cod, always changing the water. Blanch, removing skin and pimples, at a fast boil. Strain and reserve the water where the cod has been cooked.

2. Season the French fries with cod, garlic, salt and coriander. On top of that, put a saucepan with olive oil and sliced onions on the fire. Add the onions, pepper, and chopped olives, skinless and seedless. Mix in the cod, tomato extract, coconut milk, and a little water to prepare the cod. Let them all cook a lot. There was a lot of sauce moving on. Get the salt tested. Sliced potatoes and carrots are cooked.

3. In a blender, whisk together milk, wheat and 2 cups milk 1 1/2 tablespoons all-purpose flour 1 tablespoon butter 1 egg 1/2 cup sour cream Nutmeg, black pepper and melted salt butter. Bring it to the fire and stir until it thickens the mixture. Finally, add the milk, nutmeg, black pepper, beaten egg and salt.

4. After rubbing a clove of garlic inside, grease a plate with olive oil. In alternate layers, arrange the cod, potato, and carrot. Cover all with sauce and bake for 20 minutes in an air fryer at 3800F.

## 70.Salmon Fillet

Preparation Time: 10 Minutes

Cooking Time: 15 Minutes

Servings: 2-4

### Ingredients:

- 1 lb salmon fillet
- Sliced pitted olives
- Oregano
- 3 tbsp. soy sauce
- Salt to taste
- Olive oil to taste
- Lemon
- Aluminum foil
- ½ sliced onion

### Directions:

1. Wash the salmon with lemon juice.

2. Heat the oil and add the sliced onion, leaving it on the fire until it becomes transparent. Reservation.

3. Cover a baking sheet with aluminum foil so that leftovers can cover all the fish.

4. In the foil on the baking sheet, place the fish already seasoned with salt, drizzle with olive oil and soy sauce.

5. Garnish with sliced olives and a little oregano. Pour the onion on top. Wrap with aluminum foil so that the liquid does not spill when it starts to heat up.

6. Bake in the air fryer at 4000F for about 30 minutes.

7. Serve with vegetables and green salad.

## 71.Hake Fillet with Potatoes

Preparation Time: 10 Minutes

Cooking Time: 30 Minutes

Servings: 2-4

### Ingredients:

- 8 fillets of hake
- 4 raw potatoes
- 1 bell pepper
- 2 tomatoes
- 1 onion Good quality tomato sauce.
- Oregano
- Oil for greasing

### Directions:

1. As desired, season the fillets and reserve for 10 minutes. Use olive oil to grease an ovenproof dish to create a coat of potato, then put the fillets on the potato. Drizzle with tomato sauce (1/2 can) and add onion, tomato, bell pepper, oregano to taste.

2. With the rest of the potatoes, seal. Cover and bake with foil until the potatoes are tender. Using lemon juice, wash the salmon. Heat the oil until it becomes transparent, and add the sliced onion, leaving it on the flames. On reservation.

3. Cover a baking sheet of aluminum foil so that all the fish can be covered with leftovers.

4. Place the fish, which is already seasoned with salt in the foil on the baking sheet, drizzle with olive oil and soy sauce.

5. Add chopped olives and a little oregano to the garnish. On top, pour the onion. Wrap the aluminum foil so that as it begins to heat up, the liquid does not leak.

6. Bake in an air-fryer for about 30 minutes at 4000F. 7. Serve with green salad and vegetables.

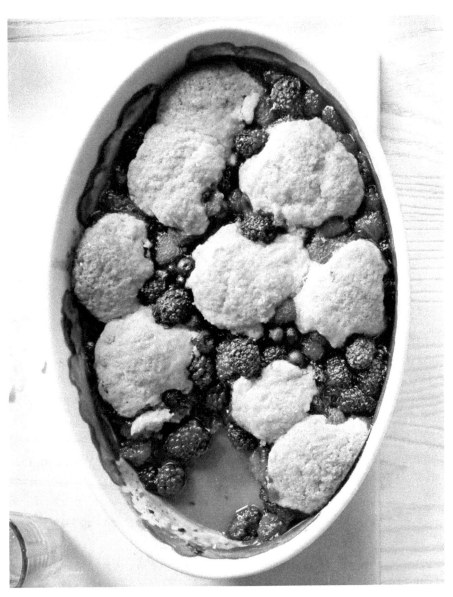

### 72.Delicious Raspberry Cobbler

Total time: 20 min

Prep time: 10 min

Cook time: 10 min

Yield: 6 serving

**Ingredients:**

- 1 egg, lightly beaten
- 1 cup raspberries, sliced
- 2 tsp. swerve
- 1/2 tsp. vanilla
- 1 tbsp. butter, melted
- 1 cup almond flour

**Directions:**

1. Place the Cuisinart oven in place 1. With the rack.
2. To the baking dish, add the raspberries.
3. Sprinkle with raspberries and sweetener.
4. In a dish, combine the almond flour, vanilla, and butter together.
5. Apply the egg to the mixture of almond flour and whisk well to blend.
6. Spread a mixture of almond flour over the sliced raspberries.
7. Set for 15 minutes to bake at 350 f. Place the baking dish in the preheated oven after five minutes.
8. Enjoy and serve.

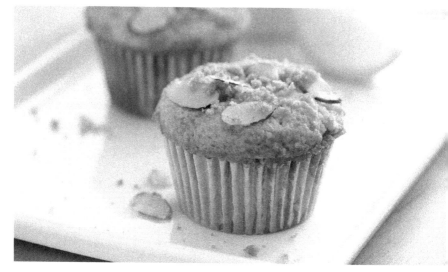

## 73.Orange Almond Muffins

Total time: 30 min

Prep time: 10 min

Cook time: 25 min

Yield: 2 servings

Ingredients:

- 4 eggs
- 1 tsp. baking soda
- 1 orange zest
- 1 orange juice
- 1/2 cup butter, melted
- 3 cups almond flour

Directions:

1. Place the Cuisinart oven in place 1. with the rack.
2. Line and set aside 12-cups of a muffin tin with cupcake liners.
3. In a big bowl, add all the ingredients and blend until well mixed.
4. In the prepared muffin pan, pour the mixture into it.
5. Set for 25 minutes to bake at 350 f. Place the muffin tin in the preheated oven for 5 minutes.
6. Enjoy and serve.

## 74.Easy Almond Butter Pumpkin Spice Cookies

Total time: 30 min

Prep time: 10 min

Cook time:25 min

Yield: 6 servings

Ingredients:

- 1/4 tsp. pumpkin pie spice
- 1 tsp. liquid Stevie
- 6 oz. almond butter
- 1/3 cup pumpkin puree

**Directions:**

1. Place the Cuisinart oven in place 1. with the rack.

2. In the food processor, add all ingredients and process until simply combined.

3. Into the parchment-lined baking tray, drop spoonsful of mixture.

4. Set to bake for 23 minutes at 350 f. Place the baking pan in the preheated oven after five minutes.

5. Enjoy and serve.

## 75.Moist Pound Cake

Total time: 40 min

Prep time: 15 min

Cook time: 25 min

Yield: 2 serving

**Ingredients:**

- 4 eggs
- 1 cup almond flour
- 1/2 cup sour cream
- 1 tsp. vanilla
- 1 cup monk fruit sweetener
- 1/4 cup cream cheese
- 1/4 cup butter
- 1 tsp. baking powder
- 1 tbsp. coconut flour

**Directions:**

1. Place the Cuisinart oven in place 1. With the rack.

2. Mix the almond flour, baking powder, and coconut flour together in a big bowl.

3. Add the cream cheese and butter to a separate bowl and microwave for 30 seconds. Stir well, then microwave for 30 more seconds.

4. Stir in the sour cream, sweetener, and vanilla. Only stir well.

5. Pour the mixture of cream cheese into the almond flour mixture and whisk until mixed.

6. Add the eggs one by one to the batter and stir until well mixed.

7. Pour the batter into a cake pan of prepared oil.

8. Set to bake for 60 minutes at 350 f. Place the cake pans in the preheated oven after five minutes.

9. Slicing and serving.

## 76.Banana Butter Brownie

Total time: 25 min

Prep time: 10 min

Cook time: 15 min

Yield: 6 serving

### Ingredients:

- 1 scoop protein powder
- 2 tbsp. cocoa powder
- 1 cup bananas, overripe
- 1/2 cup almond butter, melted

### Directions:

1. Place the Cuisinart oven in place 1. with the rack.

2. In the blender, add all the ingredients and blend until smooth.

3. Fill the greased cake pan with batter.

4. Set for 21 minutes to bake at 325 f. Place the cake pans in the preheated oven after five minutes.

5. Enjoy and serve.

## 77.Peanut Butter Muffins

Total time: 10 min

Prep time: 15 min

Cook time: 15 min

Yield: 12 serving

**Ingredients:**

- 1 cup peanut butter
- 1/2 cup maple syrup
- 1/2 cup of cocoa powder
- 1 cup applesauce
- 1 tsp. baking soda
- 1 tsp. vanilla

**Directions:**

1. Place the Cuisinart oven in place 1. with the rack.
2. Line and set aside 12-cups of a muffin tin with cupcake liners.
3. In the blender, add all the ingredients and blend until smooth.
4. Pour the blended mixture into the muffin tin you have packed.
5. Set for 25 minutes to bake at 350 f. Place the muffin tin in the preheated oven for 5 minutes.
6. Enjoy and serve.

## 78.Baked Apple Slices

Total time: 40 min

Prep time: 15 min

Cook time: 25 min

Yield: 6 serving

**Ingredients:**

- 2 apples, peel, core, and slice
- 1 tsp. cinnamon
- 2 tbsp. butter
- 1/4 cup of sugar
- 1/4 cup brown sugar
- 1/4 tsp. salt

**Directions:**

1. Place the Cuisinart oven in place 1. with the rack.

2. In the zip-lock container, add cinnamon, sugar, brown sugar, and salt and combine well.

3. Fill the bag with apple slices and shake until well coated.

4. Apply the apple slices to the greased 9-inch baking dish.

5. Set to bake for 35 minutes at 350 f. Place the baking dish in the preheated oven after five minutes.

6. Enjoy and serve.

## 79.Vanilla Peanut Butter Cake

Total time: 40 min

Prep time: 15 min

Cook time: 25 min

Yield: 8 serving

**Ingredients:**

- 1 1/2 cups all-purpose flour
- 1/3 cup vegetable oil
- 1 tsp. baking soda
- 1/2 cup peanut butter powder
- 1 tsp. vanilla
- 1 tbsp. apple cider vinegar
- 1 cup of water
- 1 cup of sugar
- 1/2 tsp. salt

**Directions:**

1. Place the Cuisinart oven in place 1. with the rack.

2. Mix the flour, baking soda, peanut butter powder, sugar and salt together in a large mixing bowl.

3. Whisk the oil, vanilla, vinegar, and water together in a small cup.

4. Pour the mixture of oil into the mixture of flour and whisk until well mixed.

5. Fill the greased cake pan with batter.

6. Set to bake for 35 minutes at 350 f. Place the cake pans in the preheated oven after five minutes

7. Cut and serve.

## 80.Moist Chocolate Brownies

Total time: 25 min

Prep time: 10 min

Cook time: 15 min

Yield: 6 serving

### Ingredients:

- 1 1/3 cups all-purpose flour
- 1/2 tsp. baking powder
- 1/3 cup cocoa powder
- 1 cup of sugar
- 1/2 tsp. vanilla
- 1/2 cup vegetable oil
- 1/2 cup water
- 1/2 tsp. salt

### Directions:

1. Place the cuisine-style oven with the rack in place 1.

2. Mix the flour, baking powder, cocoa powder, sugar and salt together in a large mixing bowl.

3. Whisk the oil, water and vanilla together in a small cup.

4. Pour the mixture of oil into the flour and blend until well mixed.

5. Pour in the greased baking dish with the batter.

6. Set to bake for 25 minutes at 350 f. Place the baking sheet in the preheated oven after five minutes.

7. Cut and serve.

## 81.Yummy Scalloped Pineapple

Total time: 40 min

Prep time: 10 min

Cook time: 25 min

Yield: 6 serving

## Ingredients:

- 3 eggs, lightly beaten
- 8 oz. can crush pineapple, un-drained
- 2 cups of sugar
- 4 cups of bread cubes
- 1/4 cup milk
- 1/2 cup butter, melted

## Directions:

1. Place the Cuisinart oven in place 1. with the rack.
2. Mix the eggs with the milk, butter, crushed pineapple, and sugar in a mixing cup.
3. To coat, add bread cubes and stir well.
4. Move the mixture to a greased dish for baking.
5. Set to bake for 40 minutes at 350 f. Place the baking dish in the preheated oven after five minutes.
6. Enjoy and serve.

## 82.Vanilla Lemon Cupcakes

Total time: 25 min

Prep time: 10 min

Cook time: 15 min

Yield: 6 serving

## Ingredients:

- 1 egg
- 1/2 cup milk
- 2 tbsp. canola oil
- 1/4 tsp. baking soda
- 3/4 tsp. baking powder
- 1 tsp. lemon zest, grated
- 1/2 cup sugar
- 1 cup flour
- 1/2 tsp. vanilla
- 1/2 tsp. salt

## Directions:

1. Place the Cuisinart oven in place 1. with the rack.
2. Line and set aside 12-cups of a muffin tin with cupcake liners.
3. Whisk the egg, vanilla, milk, oil, and sugar together in a bowl until smooth.
4. Apply the remaining ingredients and combine until mixed.
5. Load the batter into the muffin tin that has been packed.
6. Set for 20 minutes to bake at 350 f. Place the muffin tin in the preheated oven for 5 minutes.
7. Enjoy and serve.

## 83. Walnut Carrot Cake

Total time: 25 min

Prep time: 10 min

Cook time: 15 min

Yield: 4 serving

## Ingredients:

- 1 egg
- 1/2 cup sugar

- 1/4 cup canola oil
- 1/4 cup walnuts, chopped
- 1/2 tsp. baking powder
- 1/2 cup flour
- 1/4 cup grated carrot
- 1/2 tsp. vanilla
- 1/2 tsp. cinnamon

**Directions:**

1. Place the Cuisinart oven in place 1. with the rack.
2. Beat the sugar and oil in a medium bowl for 1 minute. Apply the vanilla, egg and cinnamon and beat for 30 seconds.
3. Apply the remaining ingredients and stir well until mixed.
4. Pour the batter into the baking bowl, which is greased.
5. Set for 30 minutes to bake at 350 f. Place the baking dish in the preheated oven after five minutes.
6. Enjoy and serve.

## 84.Baked Peaches

Total time: 40 min

Prep time: 10 min

Cook time: 25 min

Yield: 6 serving

**Ingredients:**

- 4 freestone peaches, cut in half and remove stones
- 2 tbsp. sugar
- 8 tsp. brown sugar
- 1 tsp. cinnamon
- 4 tbsp. butter, cut into pieces

**Directions:**

1. Place the Cuisinart oven in place 1. with the rack.

2. In a baking dish, put the peach halves and fill each half with 1 tsp. of brown sugar.

3. Place butter on top of the halves of each peach.

4. Mix the cinnamon and sugar together and drizzle over the peaches.

5. Set for 30 minutes to bake at 375 f. Place the baking dish in the preheated oven after five minutes.

6. Enjoy and serve.

## 85.Cinnamon Apple Crisp

Total time: 35 min

Prep time: 10 min

Cook time: 20 min

Yield: 4 serving

**Ingredients:**

- 1/8 tsp. ground clove
- 1/8 tsp. ground nutmeg
- 2 tbsp. honey
- 4 1/2 cups apples, diced
- 1 tsp. ground cinnamon
- 1 tbsp. cornstarch
- 1 tsp. vanilla
- 1/2 lemon juice
- For topping:
- 1 cup rolled oats
- 1/3 cup coconut oil, melted
- 1 tsp. cinnamon
- 1/3 cup honey
- 1/2 cup almond flour

**Directions:**

1. Place the Cuisinart oven in place 1. with the rack.

2. Mix the apples, vanilla, lemon juice, and honey in a medium-sized dish. Sprinkle it on top of herbs and cornstarch and stir well.

3. Load the combination of apples into the greased baking bowl.

4. Mix together the coconut oil, cinnamon, almond flour, oats and honey in a small bowl and scatter over the apple mixture.

5. Set to bake for 40 minutes at 350 f. Place the baking dish in the preheated oven after five minutes.

6. Enjoy and serve.

## 86.Apple Cake

Total time: 35 min

Prep time: 15 min

Cook time: 20 min

Yield: 12 serving

**Ingredients:**

- 2 cups apples, peeled and chopped
- 1/4 cup sugar
- 1/4 cup butter, melted
- 12 oz. apple juice
- 3 cups all-purpose flour
- 3 tsp. baking powder
- 1 1/2 tbsp. ground cinnamon
- 1 tsp. salt

**Directions:**

1. Place the Cuisinart oven in place 1. with the rack.

2. Mix the rice, salt, sugar, cinnamon, and baking powder together in a big dish.

3. Mix until well mixed, add melted butter and apple juice and mix.

4. Attach apples and fold thoroughly.

5. Pour the batter into the baking bowl, which is greased.

6. Set for 45 minutes to bake at 350 f. Place the baking dish in the preheated oven after five minutes.

7. Enjoy and serve.

## 87.Almond Cranberry Muffins

Total time: 35 min

Prep time: 15 min

Cook time: 20 min

Yield: 6 serving

### Ingredients:

- 2 eggs
- 1 tsp. vanilla
- 1/4 cup sour cream
- 1/2 cup cranberries
- 1 1/2 cups almond flour
- 1/4 tsp. cinnamon
- 1 tsp. baking powder
- 1/4 cup swerve
- Pinch of salt

### Directions:

1. Place the Cuisinart oven in place 1. with the rack.

2. Set aside and line 6-cups of a muffin tin with cupcake liners.

3. Put the sour cream, vanilla, and eggs in a cup.

4. Attach the remaining ingredients and beat until smooth, save for the cranberries.

5. Remove cranberries and fold thoroughly.

6. Load the batter into the muffin tin that has been packed.

7. Set for 30 minutes to bake at 325 f. Place the muffin tin in the preheated oven for 5 minutes.

8. Enjoy and serve.

## 88.Vanilla Butter Cake

Total time: 30 min

Prep time: 10 min

Cook time: 20 min

Yield: 8 serving

### Ingredients:

- 1 egg, beaten
- 1/2 tsp. vanilla
- 3/4 cup sugar
- 1 cup all-purpose flour
- 1/2 cup butter, softened

### Directions:

1. Place the cuisine-style oven with the rack in place 1.
2. Mix the sugar and butter together in a mixing cup.
3. Apply the egg, rice, and vanilla and whisk until mixed together.
4. Pour in the greased baking dish with the batter.
5. Set for 35 minutes to bake at 350 f. Place the baking sheet in the preheated oven after five minutes.
6. Cut and eat.

## 89.Coconut Butter Apple Bars

Total time: 40 min

Prep time: 10 min

Cook time: 30 min

Yield: 8 serving

### Ingredients:

- 1 tbsp. ground flax seed

- 1/4 cup coconut butter, softened
- 1 cup pecans
- 1 cup of water
- 1/4 cup dried apples
- 1 1/2 tsp. baking powder
- 1 1/2 tsp. cinnamon
- 1 tsp. vanilla
- 2 tbsp. swerve

## Directions:

1. Place the cuisine-style oven with the rack in place 1.
2. In the blender, add all of the ingredients and blend until smooth.
3. Pour the mixed mixture into the baking dish with oil.
4. Set to bake for 50 minutes at 350 f. Place the baking sheet in the preheated oven after five minutes.
5. Cut and eat.

## 90.Easy Blueberry Muffins

Total time: 40 min

Prep time: 10 min

Cook time: 30 min

Yield: 8 serving

## Ingredients:

- o  oz. plain yogurt
- ½ cup fresh blueberries
- 2 tsp. baking powder, gluten-free
- ¼ cup swerve
- 2 ½ cups almond flour
- ½ tsp. vanilla
- 3 eggs

- Pinch of salt

## Directions:

1. Place the Cuisinart oven in place 1. with the rack.

2. Set aside and line 6-cups of a muffin tin with cupcake liners.

3. Mix the egg, yogurt, vanilla, and salt in a bowl until smooth.

4. Add the flour, swerve and baking powder, and mix until smooth again.

5. Add the blueberries and blend well with them.

6. Load the batter into the muffin tin that has been packed.

7. Placed to bake for 35 minutes at 325 f. Place the muffin tin in the preheated oven for 5 minutes.

8. Enjoy and serve.

## 91.Tasty Almond Macaroons

Total time: 20 min

Prep time: 10 min

Cook time: 10 min

Yield: 12 serving

## Ingredients:

- 2 egg whites
- 10 oz. almonds, sliced
- 1/2 tsp. vanilla extract
- 3/4 cup Splenda

## Directions:

1. Place the Cuisinart oven in place 1. with the rack.

2. Beat the egg whites in a bowl until foamy, then add the Splenda and vanilla and mix until low.

3. Apply the egg mixture to the almonds and fold softly.

4. Slip the mixture into the parchment-lined baking pan using a spoon.

5. Set for 15 minutes to bake at 350 f. Place the baking pan in the preheated oven after five minutes.

6. Enjoy and serve.

## 92.Moist Baked Donuts

Total time: 20 min

Prep time: 10 min

Cook time: 10 min

Yield: 12 serving

**Ingredients:**

- 2 eggs
- 3/4 cup sugar
- 1/2 cup buttermilk
- 1/4 cup vegetable oil
- 1 cup all-purpose flour
- 1/2 tsp. vanilla
- 1 tsp. baking powder
- 1/2 tsp. salt

**Directions:**

1. Place the Cuisinart oven in place 1. with the rack.
2. Spray the donut pan and set it aside with the cooking spray.
3. Mix the oil, vanilla, baking powder, sugar, eggs, buttermilk, and salt together in a bowl until well mixed.
4. Stir in the flour and blend until the mixture is tender.
5. Load the batter into the donut pan that has been packed.
6. Set for 20 minutes to bake at 350 f. Place the donut pans in the preheated oven after five minutes.
7. Enjoy and serve.

## 93.Eggless Brownies

Total time: 40 min

Prep time: 10 min

Cook time: 30 min

Yield: 12 serving

Ingredients:

- 1/4 cup walnuts, chopped
- 1/3 cup cocoa powder
- 2 tsp. baking powder
- 1 cup of sugar
- 1 cup all-purpose flour
- 1/2 cup chocolate chips
- 2 tsp. vanilla
- 1 tbsp. milk
- 3/4 cup yogurt
- 1/2 cup butter, melted
- 1/4 tsp. salt

Directions:

1. Place the cuisine-style oven with the rack in place 1.
2. Sift the rice, chocolate powder, baking powder and salt into a large mixing cup. Mix and put aside well.
3. Add the sugar, vanilla, cream, and yogurt to another dish, and whisk until well mixed.
4. Apply the flour mixture to the mixture of butter and combine until just blended.
5. Fold in some chocolate chips and walnuts.
6. Pour the batter into a baking dish that has been packed.
7. Set to bake for 45 minutes at 350 f. Place the baking sheet in the preheated oven after five minutes.
8. Cut and eat.

## 94.Vanilla Banana Brownies

Total time: 40 min

Prep time: 10 min

Cook time: 30 min

Yield: 12 serving

**Ingredients:**

- 1 egg
- 1 cup all-purpose flour
- 4 oz. white chocolate
- 1/4 cup butter
- 1 tsp. vanilla extract
- 1/2 cup granulated sugar
- 2 medium bananas, mashed
- 1/4 tsp. salt

**Directions:**

1. Place the cuisine-style oven with the rack in place 1.
2. In a microwave-safe mug, add white chocolate and butter, and microwave for 30 seconds. Stir until it melts.
3. Send sugar a stir. Add mashed bananas, vanilla, eggs, and salt and combine until mixed together.
4. Attach rice, then blend until just blended together.
5. Pour in the greased baking dish with the batter.
6. Placed to bake for 25 minutes at 350 f. Place the baking sheet in the preheated oven after five minutes.
7. Cut and eat.

**95.Choco Cookies**

Total time: 20 min

Prep time: 10 min

Cook time: 10 min

Yield: 12 serving

**Ingredients:**

- 3 egg whites
- 3/4 cup cocoa powder, unsweetened
- 1 3/4 cup confectioner sugar
- 1 1/2 tsp. vanilla

**Directions:**

1. Place the Cuisinart oven in place 1. with the rack.
2. Whip the egg whites in a mixing bowl until the soft peaks are fluffy. Add the chocolate, cinnamon, and vanilla slowly.
3. Drop the teaspoonful into 32 tiny cookies on a parchment-lined baking pan.
4. Set for 8 minutes to bake at 350 f. Place the baking pan in the preheated oven after five minutes.
5. Enjoy and serve.

## 96.Chocolate Chip Cookies

Total time: 20 min

Prep time: 10 min

Cook time: 10 min

Yield: 30 serving

**Ingredients:**

- 1 egg
- 2/3 cup sugar
- 1 tsp. vanilla
- 1 cup butter, softened
- 12 oz. chocolate chips
- 2 cups self-rising flour
- 1/2 cup brown sugar

**Directions:**

1. Place the Cuisinart oven in place 1. with the rack.

2. In a broad mixing cup, add the sugar, vanilla, and egg and beat until mixed.

3. Apply the brown sugar and sugar and mix until smooth.

4. Add the flour slowly and stir until just mixed.

5. Fold the chocolate chips together.

6. Spoon the cookie dough balls into a baking tray lined with parchment.

7. Set for 15 minutes to bake at 375 f. Place the baking pan in the preheated oven after five minutes.

8. Enjoy and serve.

## 97.Oatmeal Cake

Total time: 40 min

Prep time: 10 min

Cook time: 30 min

Yield: 8 serving

### Ingredients:

- 2 eggs, beaten
- 1 tbsp. cocoa powder
- 1/2 tsp. salt
- 1 tsp. baking soda
- 1/2 cup butter, softened
- 1 cup granulated sugar
- 1 cup brown sugar
- 1 3/4 cups flour
- 1 cup quick oats
- 3/4 cup mix nuts, chopped
- 2 cups chocolate chips
- 1 3/4 cup boiling water

### Directions:

1. Place the cuisine-style oven with the rack in place 1.

2. Combine the boiling water in a large bowl with the oats.

3. Stir in the butter and sugar before the butter has melted.

4. Combine the rice, baking soda, cinnamon, cocoa powder, 1 cup of chocolate chips, half the diced nuts, and the egg. Mix once combined.

5. Sprinkle the remaining nuts and chocolate chips over the top of the cake batter and add the batter into the greased cake tin.

6. Set to bake for 45 minutes at 350 f. Place the baking sheet in the preheated oven after five minutes.

7. Cut and eat.

## 98.Delicious Banana Cake

Total time: 50 min

Prep time: 10 min

Cook time: 40 min

Yield: 8 serving

### Ingredients:

- 2 large eggs, beaten
- 1 tsp. baking powder
- 1 1/2 cup sugar, granulated
- 1 tsp. vanilla extract
- 1/2 cup butter
- 1 cup milk
- 2 cups all-purpose flour
- 2 bananas, mashed
- 1 tsp. baking soda

### Directions:

1. Place the cuisine-style oven with the rack in place 1.

2. Beat the sugar and butter together in a mixing bowl until smooth. Beaten eggs are inserted to blend properly.

3. Apply to the mixture the milk, vanilla extract, baking soda, baking powder, flour, and mashed bananas, and beat for 2 minutes. Mix thoroughly.

4. Pour in the greased baking dish with the batter.

5. Set to bake for 45 minutes at 350 f. Place the baking sheet in the preheated oven after five minutes.

6. Slice and eat.

## 99. Chocolate Cake

Total time: 50 min

Prep time: 10 min

Cook time: 40 min

Yield: 8 serving

### Ingredients:

- 1/2 cup warm water
- 2 3/4 cups flour
- 1 cup buttermilk
- 1 cup shortening
- 1 cup sugar, granulated
- 1 cup brown sugar
- 2 large eggs
- 1/2 cup cocoa powder
- 1 tsp. baking soda

### Directions:

1. Place the cuisine-style oven with the rack in place 1.

2. Beat together powdered sugar, granulated sugar and shortening until smooth in a large mixing cup.

3. Mix well with the eggs, cocoa powder, rice, and buttermilk when combined.

4. In warm water, dissolve the soda and stir into the batter.

5. Pour in the greased baking dish with the batter.

6. Set for 35 minutes to bake at 350 f. Place the baking sheet in the preheated oven after five minutes.

7. Slice and eat.

## 100.Almond Blueberry Bars

Total time: 60 min

Prep time: 10 min

Cook time: 40 min

Yield: 8 serving

### Ingredients:

- 1/4 cup blueberries
- 3 tbsp. coconut oil
- 2 tbsp. coconut flour
- 1/2 cup almond flour
- 3 tbsp. water
- 1 tbsp. chia seeds
- 1 tsp. vanilla
- 1 tsp. fresh lemon juice
- 2 tbsp. erythritol
- 1/4 cup almonds, sliced
- 1/4 cup coconut flakes

### Directions:

1. Place the Cuisinart oven with the rack in place 1.

2. Line a baking dish and set it aside with parchment paper.

3. Mix the water and the chia seeds together in a shallow cup. Put back aside.

4. In a tub, mix all of the ingredients together. Attach a blend of chia and whisk well.

5. Pour the mixture into the baking dish prepared and spread uniformly.

6.  Set to bake for 55 minutes, at 300 f. Place the baking dish in the preheated oven after five minutes.

7.  Slice and eat.

# Conclusion

What is so unique about air frying, though? In a fraction of the time, the air fryer will replace your refrigerator, your fridge, your deep fryer, and your dehydrator, and cook tasty meals uniformly. The air fryer is a game changer if you're trying to supply your family with nutritious meals, just don't have a lot of time. This book is a compilation of 100 amazing and palatable air fryer recipes that you must give a try.

# The Affordable Air Fryer Cookbook

**The Ultimate Guide with 100 Quick and Delicious Affordable Recipes for beginners**

*By Marisa Smith*

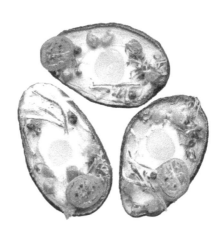

## Introduction

We all love the deep-fried food taste, but not the calories or hassle of frying in too much fat. To solve this issue, the Air fryer was designed as its revolutionary nature allows you to cook food while frying with one or two tablespoons of oil and remove extra fat from the meal. This recipe book includes some of the amazing recipes that your Air fryer can prepare. From French fries to spring rolls and even soufflés, the choices are limitless!

# Air Fryer Recipes

## 1. Chewy Breakfast Brownies

Total time: 40 min

Prep time: 10 min

Cook time: 30 min

Yield: 9 servings

### Ingredients:

- 1 egg
- 2 tbsp. cocoa powder
- 1 tsp. vanilla
- 1 1/4 cup milk
- 1/2 cup applesauce
- 1/4 cup brown sugar
- 2 1/4 cup quick oats

### Directions:

1. Spray and set aside a 9*9-inch baking dish with cooking spray.

2. Insert a rack of wire in rack position 6. Pick bake, set temperature to 350 f, 30-minute timer. To preheat the oven, press start.

3. Mix brown sugar, cocoa powder, and oats together in a big cup.

4. Add wet ingredients: blend until well mixed.

5. Pour the baking dish with the mixture and spread it properly.

6. Place foil on the baking dish and bake for 15 minutes. After 15 minutes, remove the cover and bake for 15 more minutes.

7. Enjoy and serve.

## 2.Peach Banana Baked Oatmeal

Total time: 45 min

Prep time: 10 min

Cook time: 35 min

Yield: 5 servings

### Ingredients:

- Two eggs
- 1 tsp. vanilla
- 1 1/2 cups milk
- 1/2 tsp. cinnamon
- 3/4 tsp. baking powder
- 1/4 cup ground flax seed
- 2 1/2 cups steel-cut oats
- 2 bananas, sliced
- 1 peach, sliced
- 1/2 tsp. salt

### Directions:

1. Spray an 8*8-inch baking dish with cooking spray and set aside.
2. Insert wire rack in rack position 6. Select bake, set temperature 350 f, timer for 35 minutes. Press start to preheat the oven.
3. Add all ingredients except one banana into the mixing bowl and mix until well combined.
4. Pour mixture into the baking dish and spread well. Spread the remaining 1 banana slices on top and bake for 35 minutes.
5. Serv e and enjoy.

### 3.Healthy Poppy seed Baked Oatmeal

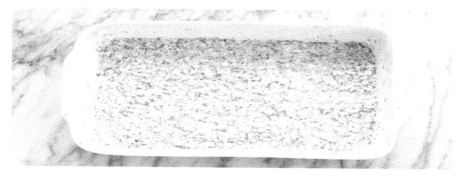

Total time: 35 min

Prep time: 10 min

Cook time: 25 min

Yield: 8 servings

**Ingredients:**

- 3 eggs
- 1 tbsp. poppy seeds
- 1 tsp. baking powder
- 1 tsp. vanilla
- 1 tsp. lemon zest
- 1/4 cup lemon juice
- 1/4 cup honey
- 2 cups almond milk
- 3 cups rolled oats
- 1/4 tsp. salt

**Directions:**

1. Spray a baking dish with cooking spray and set it aside.

2. Insert wire rack in rack position 6. Select bake, set temperature 350 f, timer for 25 minutes. Press start to preheat the oven.

3. In a large bowl, mix together all ingredients: until well combined.

4. Pour mixture into the baking dish and spread well, and bake for 25 minutes.

5. Serve and enjoy.

## 4.Healthy Berry Baked Oatmeal

Total time: 30 min

Prep time: 10 min

Cook time: 20 min

Yield: 4 servings

### Ingredients:

- 1 egg
- 1 cup blueberries
- 1/2 cup blackberries
- 1/2 cup strawberries, sliced
- 1/4 cup maple syrup
- 1 1/2 cups milk
- 1 1/2 tsp. baking powder
- 2 cups old fashioned oats
- 1/2 tsp. salt

### Directions:

1. Spray with cooking spray on a baking dish and put aside.

2. Insert a rack of wire in rack position 6. Pick bake, set temperature to 375 f, 20 minute timer. To preheat the oven, press start.

3. Blend together the peas, salt and baking powder in a mixing cup. Stir well and Mix vanilla, egg, maple syrup, and tea.

4. Add berries and blend well with them. Into the baking bowl, add the mixture and bake for 20 minutes.

5. Enjoy and serve.

## 5.Apple Oatmeal Bars

Total time: 35 min

Prep time: 10 min

Cook time: 25 min

Yield: 12 servings

## Ingredients:

- 2 eggs
- 2 tbsp. butter
- 2 tsp. baking powder
- 2 cups apple, chopped
- 3 cups old fashioned oats
- Pinch of salt
- 1/2 cup honey
- 1 tbsp. vanilla
- 1 cup milk
- 1 tbsp. cinnamon

## Directions:

1. Spray a 9*13-inch baking dish with cooking spray and set aside.
2. Insert wire rack in rack position 6. Select bake, set temperature 375 f, timer for 25 minutes. Press start to preheat the oven.
3. In a mixing bowl, mix together dry ingredients.
4. In a separate bowl, whisk together wet ingredients. Pour wet ingredient mixture into the dry mixture and mix well.
5. Pour mixture into the baking dish and bake for 25 minutes.
6. Slice and serve.

## 6.Walnut Banana Bread

Prep time: 10 minutes

Cook time: 50 minutes

Yield: 10 servings

**Ingredients:**

- 3 eggs
- 1 tsp. baking soda
- 4 tbsp. olive oil
- 1/2 cup walnuts, chopped
- 2 cups almond flour
- 3 bananas

**Directions:**

1. Grease loaf pan with butter and set aside.
2. Insert wire rack in rack position 6. Select bake, set temperature 350 f, timer for 50 minutes. Press start to preheat the oven.
3. Add all ingredients into the food processor and process until combined.
4. Pour batter into the prepared loaf pan and bake for 50 minutes.
5. Slices and serve.

## 7.Cinnamon Zucchini Bread

Total time: 1 hour 10 min

Prep time: 10 min

Cook time: 60 min

Yield: 12 servings

**Ingredients:**

- 3 eggs
- 1/2 tsp. nutmeg
- 1 1/2 tsp. baking powder
- 1 1/2 tsp. erythritol
- 2 1/2 cups almond flour
- 1 tsp. vanilla

- 1/2 cup walnuts, chopped
- 1 cup zucchini, grated & squeeze out all liquid
- 1/4 tsp. ground ginger
- 1 tsp. cinnamon
- 1/2 cup olive oil
- 1/2 tsp. salt

## Directions:

1. Grease loaf pan with butter and set aside.
2. Insert wire rack in rack position 6. Select bake, set temperature 350 f, timer for 60 minutes. Press start to preheat the oven.
3. In a bowl, whisk eggs, vanilla, and oil. Set aside.
4. In a separate bowl, mix together almond flour, ginger, cinnamon, nutmeg, baking powder, salt, and sweetener. Set aside.
5. Add grated zucchini into the egg mixture and stir well.
6. Add dry ingredients into the egg mixture and stir to combine.
7. Pour batter into the loaf pan and bake for 60 minutes.
8. Slices and serve.

## 8. Italian Breakfast Bread

Total time: 60 min

Prep time: 10 min

Cook time: 50 min

Yield: 10 servings

## Ingredients:

- 1/2 cup black olives, chopped
- 5 sun-dried tomatoes, chopped
- 2 tbsp. psyllium husk powder
- 5 egg whites
- 2 egg yolks
- 4 tbsp. coconut oil

- 2 cups flaxseed flour
- 2 tbsp. apple cider vinegar
- 1 tbsp. thyme, dried
- 1 tbsp. oregano, dried
- 2 1/2 oz. feta cheese
- 1 tbsp. baking powder
- 1/2 cup boiling water
- 1/2 tsp. salt

**Directions:**

1. Grease loaf pan with butter and set aside.
2. Insert wire rack in rack position 6. Select bake, set temperature 350 f, timer for 50 minutes. Press start to preheat the oven.
3. In a bowl, mix together psyllium husk powder, baking powder, and flaxseed.
4. Add oil and eggs and stir to combine. Add vinegar and stir well.
5. Add boiling water and stir to combine.
6. Add tomatoes, olives, and feta cheese. Mix well.
7. Pour batter into the loaf pan and bake for 50 minutes.
8. Sliced and serve.

## 9.Coconut Zucchini Bread

Total time: 55 min

Prep time: 10 min

Cook time: 45 min

Yield: 12 servings

**Ingredients:**

- 1 banana, mashed
- 1 tsp. stevia
- 4 eggs
- 1/2 cup coconut flour

- 1 tbsp. coconut oil
- 1 cup zucchini, shredded and squeeze out all liquid
- 1/2 cup walnuts, chopped
- 1 tbsp. cinnamon
- 3/4 tsp. baking soda
- 1/2 tsp. salt
- 1 tsp. apple cider vinegar
- 1/2 tsp. nutmeg

## Directions:

1. Grease the loaf pan and set it aside with butter.
2. Wire rack insertion at rack position 6. Pick bake, set temperature to 350 f, 45 minute timer. To preheat the oven, press start.
3. Whisk the egg, banana, oil and stevia together in a big mug.
4. Stir well and add all the dried ingredients, vinegar, and zucchini. Combine the walnuts and stir.
5. Through the loaf tin, add the batter and bake for 45 minutes.
6. Slicing and cooking.

## 10.Protein Banana Bread

Total time: 1 hour 20 min

Prep time: 10 min

Cook time: 1 hour 10 min

Yield: 16 servings

## Ingredients:

- 3 eggs
- 1/3 cup coconut flour
- 1/2 cup swerve
- 2 cups almond flour
- 1/2 cup ground chia seed

- 1/2 tsp. vanilla extract
- 4 tbsp. butter, melted
- 3/4 cup almond milk
- 1 tbsp. baking powder
- 1/3 cup protein powder
- 1/2 cup water
- 1/2 tsp. salt

**Directions:**

1. Grease the loaf pan and set it aside with butter.
2. Wire rack insertion at rack position 6. Bake selection, set temperature 325 f, 1 hour 10 minutes timer. To preheat the oven, press start.
3. Whisk the chia seed and 1/2 cup of water together in a small dish. Only put aside.
4. Mix the almond flour, baking powder, protein powder, coconut flour, sweetener, and salt together in a big cup.
5. Mix eggs, sugar, blend of chia seeds, vanilla extract and butter until well mixed.
6. In the prepared loaf tin, add the batter and bake for 1 hour and 10 minutes.
7. Slicing and serving

## 11. Easy Kale Muffins

Total time: 40 min

Prep time: 10 min

Cook time: 30 min

Yield: 8 servings

**Ingredients:**

- 6 eggs
- 1/2 cup milk
- 1/4 cup chives, chopped

- 1 cup kale, chopped
- Pepper
- Salt

## Directions:

21. Spray 8 cups muffin pan with cooking spray and set aside.
22. Insert wire rack in rack position 6. Select bake, set temperature 350 f, timer for 30 minutes. Press start to preheat the oven.
23. Add all ingredients into the mixing bowl and whisk well.
24. Pour mixture into the prepared muffin pan and bake for 30 minutes.
25. Serve and enjoy.

## 12.Mouthwatering Shredded BBQ Roast

Total time: 40 min

Prep time: 10 min

Cook time: 30 min

Yield: 8 servings

## Ingredients:

- 4 lbs. Pork roast
- 1 tsp. Garlic powder
- Salt and pepper to taste
- 1/2 cup water
- 2 can (11 oz.) Of barbecue sauce, keno unsweetened

## Directions:

1. Season the pork with garlic powder, salt and pepper, place in your instant pot.
2. Pour water and lock lid into place; set on the meat/stew, the high-pressure setting for 30 minutes.
3. When ready, use quick release - turn the valve from sealing to venting to release the pressure.
4. Remove pork in a bowl, and with two forks, shred the meat.

5. Pour BBQ sauce and stir to combine well.

6. Serve.

## 13.Sour and Spicy Spareribs

Total time: 50 min

Prep time: 15 min

Cook time: 35 min

Yield: 10 servings

### Ingredients:

- 5 lbs. Spare spareribs
- Salt and pepper to taste
- 2 tbsp. Of tallow
- 1/2 cup coconut amines (from coconut sap)
- 1/2 cup vinegar
- 2 tbsp. Worcestershire sauce, to taste
- 1 tsp. Chili powder
- 1 tsp. Garlic powder
- 1 tsp. Celery seeds

### Directions:

1. Break into similar parts the rack of ribs.

2. Season the spareribs on both sides with salt and ground pepper.

3. In your instant pot, add tallow and put the spareribs.

4. Mix all the remaining ingredients in a cup and spill over the spareribs.

5. Click the lid in place and set it to heat for 35 minutes on the manual setting.

6. Click "cancel" as the timer beeps, then flip the natural release gently for 20 minutes.

7. Open the cover and put the ribs on a serving tray.

8. Serve it hot.

## 14. Tender Pork Shoulder with Hot Peppers

Prep time: 10 minutes

Cook time: 30 minutes

Yield: 8 servings

### Ingredients:

- 3 lbs. Pork shoulder boneless
- Salt and ground black pepper to taste
- 3 tbsp. Of olive oil
- 1 large onion, chopped
- 2 cloves garlic minced
- 2 - 3 chili peppers, chopped
- 1 tsp. Ground coriander
- 1 tsp. ground cumin
- 1 ½ cups of bone broth (preferably homemade)
- 1/2 cup water

### Directions:

1. Season the salt and the pork meat with pepper.
2. Switch the instant pot on and press the button to sauté. When the term 'heat' appears on the show, add the oil and sauté for around 5 minutes with the onions and garlic.
3. Add the pork and cook on both sides for 1 - 2 minutes; turn off the sauté button.
4. In an instant kettle, add all the remaining ingredients.
5. Click the lid in place and set it on high heat for 30 minutes on the meat/stew level.
6. Click "cancel" as the timer beeps, then flip the natural release button gently for 15 minutes. Serve it warm.

## 15. Braised Sour Pork Filet

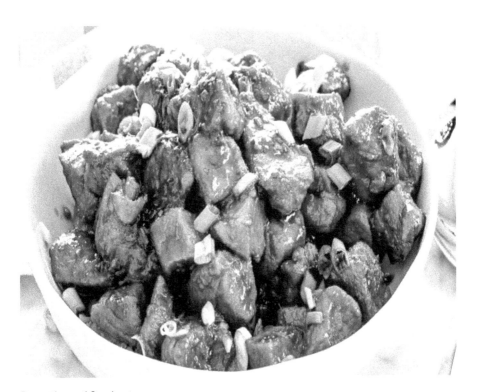

Prep time: 10 minutes

Cook time: 8 hours

Yield: 6 servings

**Ingredients:**

- 1/2 tsp. Of dry thyme
- 1/2 tsp. Of sage
- Salt and ground black pepper to taste
- 2 tabs of olive oil
- 3 lbs. Of pork fillet
- 1/3 cup of shallots (chopped)
- Three cloves of garlic (minced)
- 3/4 cup of bone broth
- 1/3 cup of apple cider vinegar

**Directions:**

1. Combine the thyme, sage, salt and black ground pepper in a shallow cup.

2. Rub the pork generously on both edges.

3. In a large frying pan, heat the olive oil and cook the pork for 2 - 3 minutes.

4. Place the pork and add the shallots and garlic in your crockpot.

5. Sprinkle with broth and apple cider vinegar/juice.

6. Cover and simmer for 8 hours on slow heat or 4-5 hours on high heat.

7. Change the salt and pepper, slice and serve with cooking juice and cut the pork from the pan.

## 16.Pork with Anise and Cumin Stir-Fry

Total time: 35 min

Prep time: 5 min

Cook time: 30 min

Yield: 4 servings

### Ingredients:

- 2 tbsp. Lard
- 2 spring onions finely chopped (only green part)
- 2 cloves garlic, finely chopped
- 2 lbs. Pork loin, boneless, cut into cubes
- Sea salt and black ground pepper to taste
- 1 green bell pepper (cut into thin strips)
- 1/2 cup water
- 1/2 tsp. Dill seeds
- 1/2 anise seeds
- 1/2 tsp. Cumin

### Directions:

1. Heat the lard n a large frying pot over medium-high heat.

2. Sauté the spring onions and garlic with a pinch of salt for 3 - 4 minutes.

3. Add the pork and simmer for about 5 - 6 minutes.

4. Add all remaining ingredients: and stir well.

5. Cover and let simmer for 15 - 20 minutes

6. Taste and adjust seasoning to taste.

7. Serve!

## 17.Baked Meatballs with Goat Cheese

Total time: 50 min

Prep time: 15 min

Cook time: 35 min

Yield: 8 servings

### Ingredients:

- 1 tbsp. Of tallow
- 2 lbs. Of ground beef
- 1 organic egg
- 1 grated onion
- 1/2 cup of almond milk (unsweetened)
- 1 cup of red wine
- 1/2 bunch of chopped parsley
- 1/2 cup of almond flour
- Salt and ground pepper to taste
- 1/2 tbsp. Of dry oregano
- 4 oz. Of hard goat cheese cut into cubes

### Directions:

1. Preheat oven to 400°f.
2. Grease a baking pan with tallow.

3. In a large bowl, combine all ingredients except goat cheese.

4. Knead the mixture until ingredients: are evenly combined.

5. Make small meatballs and place them in a prepared baking dish.

6. Place one cube of cheese on each meatball.

7. Bake for 30 - 35 minutes.

8. Serve hot.

## 18.Parisian Schnitzel

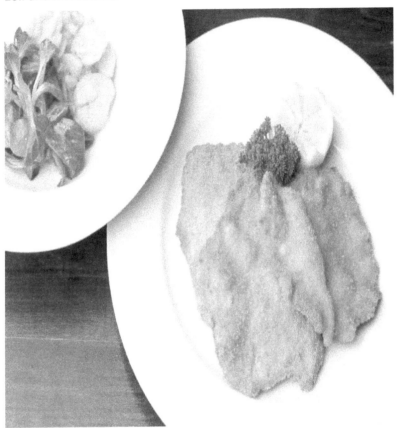

Total time: 25 min

Prep time: 15 min

Cook time: 10 min

Yield: 4 servings

**Ingredients:**

- Four veal steaks; thin schnitzel
- Salt and ground black pepper
- 2 tbsp. Of butter
- Three eggs from free-range chickens

- 4 tbsp. Of almond flour

**Directions:**

1. With salt and pepper, season the steaks.

2. Heat butter over medium heat in a large nonstick frying pan.

3. Beat the eggs in a bowl.

4. In a bowl, add the almond flour.

5. Using almond flour to roll each steak, then add and dip in the beaten eggs.

6. Fry each side for around 3 minutes.

7. Serve instantly.

### 19.Kato Beef Stroganoff

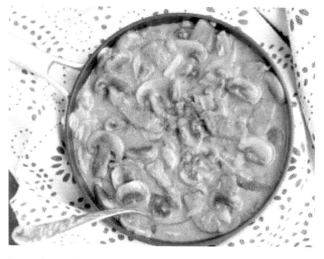

Prep time: 5 minutes

Cook time: 30 minutes

Yield: 6 servings

**Ingredients:**

- 2 lbs. Of rump or round steak or stewing steak

- 4 tbsp. Of olive oil

- 2 green onions, finely chopped

- 1 grated tomato
- 2 tbsp. Ketchup (without sugar)
- 1 cup of button mushrooms
- 1/2 cup of bone broth
- 1 cup of sour cream
- Salt and black pepper to taste

## Directions:

1. Break the beef into strips and sauté it in a large pan for frying.
2. Add the chopped onion and a pinch of salt and roast at a medium temperature for around 20 minutes.
3. Add the ketchup and mushrooms and mix for 3 - 5 minutes.
4. Pour the sour cream and bone broth and simmer for 3 to 4 minutes.
5. Remove and taste from the fire and change the salt and pepper to taste.
6. Serve it warm.

## 20.Meatloaf with Gruyere

Total time: 55 min

Prep time: 15 min

Cook time: 40 min

Yields: 6 servings

## Ingredients:

- 1 1/2 lbs. Ground beef
- 1 cup ground almonds
- 1 large egg from free-range chickens
- 1/2 cup grated gruyere cheese
- 1 tsp. Fresh parsley finely chopped
- 1 scallion finely chopped
- 1/2 tsp. Ground cumin

- 3 eggs boiled
- 2 tbsp. Of fresh grass-fed butter, melted

**Directions:**

1. Preheat the oven to 350 degrees F.

2. Combine all the ingredients in a large bowl (except for the eggs and butter).

3. Use your hands to combine the mixture properly.

4. Shape the mixture into a roll and put the sliced hard-boiled eggs in the middle.

5. To a 5x9 inch loaf pan greased with melted butter, switch the meatloaf.

6. Put in the oven and cook for 40 minutes, or until the temperature inside is 160 °F.

7. Take it out of the oven and let it sit for 10 minutes.

8. Slicing and cooking.

9.

## 21.Roasted Filet Mignon in Foil

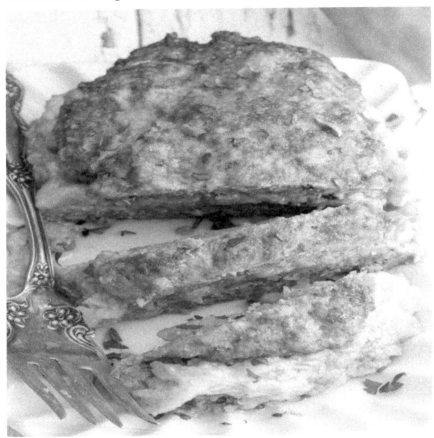

Total time: 60 min

Prep time: 15 min

Cook time: 45 min

Yield: 8 servings

**Ingredients:**

- 3 lbs. Filet mignon in one piece
- Salt to taste and ground black pepper
- 1 tsp. Of garlic powder
- 1 tsp. Of onion powder

- 1 tsp. Of cumin
- 4 tbsp. Of olive oil

**Directions:**

1. Preheat the oven to 425°f.

2. Rinse and clean the filet mignon, removing all fats, or ask your butcher to do it for you.

3. Season with salt and pepper, garlic powder, onion powder and cumin.

4. Wrap filet mignon in foil and place in a roasting pan, drizzle with the olive oil.

5. Roast for 15 minutes per pound for medium-rare or to desired doneness.

6. Remove from the oven and allow to rest for 10 -15 minutes before serving.

## 22.Stewed Beef with Green Beans

Prep time: 10 minutes

Cook time: 50 minutes

Yield: 8 servings

**Ingredients:**

- 1/2 cup olive oil
- 1 1/2 lbs. Beef cut into cubes
- 2 scallions, finely chopped
- 2 cups water
- 1 lb. Fresh green beans - trimmed and cut diagonally in half
- 1 bay leaf
- 1 grated tomato
- 1/2 cup fresh mint leaves, finely chopped
- 1 tsp. Fresh or dry rosemary
- Salt and freshly ground pepper to taste

**Directions:**

1. Chop the beef into cubes that are 1 inch thick.

2. In a big pot, heat olive oil over high heat. Sauté the beef and sprinkle it with a pinch of salt and pepper for around 4 - 5 minutes.

3. Add the scallions and mix and sauté until softened for around 3 - 4 more minutes. For 2-3 minutes, pour water and cook.

4. Add the grated tomato and bay leaf. Cook for 5 minutes or so; reduce the heat to medium-low. For about 15 minutes, cover and boil.

5. Add the rosemary, green beans, salt, fresh ground pepper and ample water to cover all the ingredients. Simmer softly, until the green beans are tender, for 15 - 20 minutes.

6. Sprinkle with the rosemary and mint, carefully blend and extract from the sun. Serve it warm.

## 23.Garlic Herb Butter Roasted Radishes

Total time: 20 min

Prep time: 10 min

Cook time: 10 min

Yield:  (4per servings)

**Ingredients:**

- 1-pound of radishes
- 2 tablespoons of unsalted butter, melted
- 1/2 teaspoon of garlic powder
- ½ teaspoon of dried parsley
- 1/4 teaspoon of dried oregano
- 1/4 teaspoon of ground black pepper

**Directions:**

1. Separate the roots from the radishes and cut them into parts.

2. Then, in a small bowl, spread butter and seasonings. Swirl the radishes in the herbal butter and place them in the Air Fryer basket.

3. Fix the temperature for 10 minutes to 350° F and adjust the timer.

4. Throw the radishes halfway through the cooking cycle in the Air Fryer basket. Enable it to cool until the edges begin to turn orange.

5. Serve it hot and drink it!

## 24.Sausage-Stuffed Mushroom Caps

Total time: 20 min

Prep time: 10 min

Cook time: 10 min

Yield: (4per servings)

### Ingredients:

- 6 large portobello mushroom caps
- ½-pound of Italian sausage
- 1/4 cup of chopped onion
- 2 tablespoons of blanched finely ground almond flour
- ¼ cup of grated Parmesan cheese
- 1 teaspoon of minced fresh garlic

### Directions:

1. To hollow each cap of the mushrooms, use a spoon and save the scraps.

2. Brown the sausage for approximately 10 minutes in a medium saucepan over medium pressure,

3. Or until completely cooked and there is no residual pink. Drain the mushroom, cabbage, almond flour, parmesan, and garlic and then add preserved scrapings. Gently fold the ingredients together and proceed to cook for another minute, then extract them from the flames.

4. Scoop the mixture equally into mushroom caps and put the caps in a bowl of 6 rounds. Place the pan in an Air Fryer basket.

5. Set the temperature to 375° F and set the eight-minute timer.

6. When frying is finished, the tops will be browned and bubbled, and serve gently.

## 25.Cheesy Cauliflower Tots

Total time: 20 min

Prep time: 10 min

Cook time: 10 min

Yield: (4per servings)

## Ingredients:

- 1 large head of cauliflower
- 1 cup of shredded mozzarella cheese
- 1/2 cup of grated Parmesan cheese
- 1large egg
- 1/4 teaspoon of garlic powder
- 1/4 teaspoon of dried parsley
- 1/8 teaspoon of onion powder

## Directions:

1. On the stovetop, fill a huge pot with 2 cups of water and place a steamer in the oven. Get the bath to a boil. Break the cauliflower into a flower and put the pot and lid on a steamer box.

2. Let the cauliflower steam for 7 minutes, until tender. Place the steamer basket in your cheesecloth or clean kitchen towel and let it cool. To remove as much excess humidity as possible, push on the sink. The mixture would be too fragile to form into tots if not all of the moisture is extracted. Mash down with a razor into a smooth consistency.

3. Place the cauliflower and add the mozzarella, parmesan, cheese, garlic powder, parsley, and onion powder in a large mixing cup. Remove before you mix properly. Smooth but easy to mold, the mix should be.

4. Roll the mixture into a tot shape by taking 2 teaspoons of the mixture. Repeat for the remaining mixture. In the Air Fryer, bring the basket in.

5. Fix the temperature for 12 minutes to 320° F and set the timer.

6. Switch the tots halfway through the cooking time. Cauliflower tots, when fully baked, should be golden. Serve it hot.

## 26.Crispy Brussels sprouts

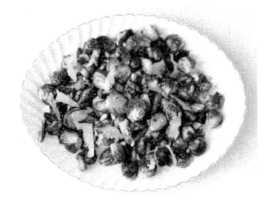

Total time: 20 min

Prep time: 10 min

Cook time: 10 min

Yield: (4per servings)

### Ingredients:

- 1-pound of Brussels sprouts
- 1 tablespoon of coconut oil
- 1 tablespoon of unsalted butter, melted

### Directions:

1. Every sprout of loose leaves from Brussels is removed and cut in half.

2. Spray it with coconut oil and drop it in the Air Fryer basket.

3. Set the temperature to 400 degrees F and for 10 minutes, change the timer. Depending on how they start browning, you might want to stir gently halfway through the cooking process.

4. When fully baked, they should be tender with darker caramelized spots. Drizzle with the molten butter and cut it out of the bowl of the fryer. Serve without hesitation.

# 27.Zucchini Parmesan Chips

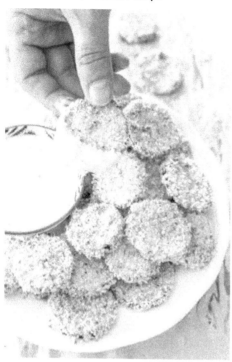

Total time: 20 min

Prep time: 10 min

Cook time: 10 min

Yield: 1 serving

## Ingredients:

- 2 medium zucchinis
- 1-ounce of pork rinds
- 1/2 cup of grated Parmesan cheese
- 1 large egg

## Directions:

1. 1/4-inch thick slices of a zucchini slice. To extract the excess moisture, place 30 minutes between two layers of paper towels or a clean kitchen towel.

2. In a food processor, put pork rinds and pulse until finely ground. Pour into a medium bowl and blend with parmesan.

3. In a small saucepan, pound the potato.

4. In the egg mixture, dip the zucchini slices and then cover as deeply as possible in the pork rind mixture. Put each slice carefully in a single layer of the Air Fryer bowl, working in batches as needed.

5. Adjust the temperature and set a 10-minute timer to 320° F.

6. Halfway into cooking time, flip chips. Serve hot and enjoy!

## 28.Roasted Garlic

Total time: 20 min

Prep time: 10 min

Cook time: 10 min

Yield: 1 serving

### Ingredients:

- 1 medium head of garlic
- 2 teaspoons of avocado oil

### Directions:

1. Strip any excess peel hanging from the garlic still cover the cloves. Shutdown 1/4 of the garlic handle, with clove tips visible.

2. Avocado oil spray. Place the garlic head in a small sheet of aluminum foil, and enclose it completely. Place it in the basket for Air Fryer.

3. Set the temperature to 400° F and change the timer for 20 minutes. If your garlic head is a little smaller, take 15 minutes to check it out.

4. Ail should be golden brown and very fluffy when finished.

5. Cloves should pop out to eat and be scattered or sliced quickly. In the refrigerator, lock in an airtight jar for up to 5 days. You can also freeze individual cloves on a baking sheet, then lock them together until frozen in a freezer-safe storage jar.

## 29.Kale Chips

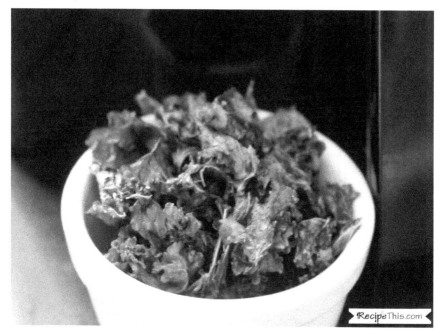

Total time: 20 min

Prep time: 10 min

Cook time: 10 min

Yield: 2 servings

### Ingredients:

- 4 cups of steamed kale
- 2 teaspoons of avocado oil
- 1/2 teaspoon of salt

### Directions:

1. Sprinkle the kale in a big bowl of avocado oil and sprinkle it with ice. Place it inside the Air Fryer basket.

2. Adjust the temperature and set a 5-minute timer to 400° f.

3. The kale will be crispy until it was done. Serve without hesitation.

## 30.Buffalo Cauliflower

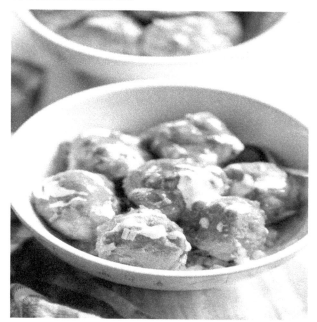

Total time: 20 min

Prep time: 10 min

Cook time: 10 min

Yield: 4 servings

**Ingredients:**

- 4 cups of cauliflower florets
- 2 tablespoons of salted butter, melted
- 1/2 (1-ounce)dry ranch seasoning packet
- 1/4 cup of buffalo sauce

**Directions:**

1. Toss the cauliflower with the butter and dry the ranch in a wide bowl. Place the basket in the Air Fryer.

2. Change the temperature and set the timer to 400°F for 5 minutes.

3. Shake the basket during the cooking process two to three times. Remove the coli flower from the fryer basket when tender and toss in the buffalo sauce. Serve it hot.

## 31.Green Bean Casserole

Total time: 20 min

Prep time: 10 min

Cook time: 10 min

Yield: 4 servings

### Ingredients:

- 4 tablespoons of unsalted butter
- 1/4 cup of diced yellow onion
- 1/2 cup of chopped white mushrooms
- 1/2 cup of heavy whipping cream
- 1 ounce of full-Fat: cream cheese
- 1/2 cup of chicken broth
- 1/4 teaspoon of xanthan gum 1-pound fresh green beans, edges trimmed
- ½ ounce of pork rinds, finely ground

### Directions:

1. Melt butter over low heat in a medium saucepan. Before they become soft and fragrant, cook the onion and mushrooms for around 3–5 minutes.

2. Add the hard whipped cream, cream cheese, and broth to the saucepan. Before, whisk quickly. Bring it to a boil, then drop it to a simmer. Sprinkle the gum with xanthan gum in the pan and fry.

3. Break the green beans into 2 parts and arrange them in a round 4-cup baking dish. Spillover those with the sauce mixture and stir until fried. With the rinds of the ground pork, fill the dish.

4. Fix the temperature to 320 degrees F and for 15 minutes, set the timer.

5. Top fork-tender when fully fried, golden and green beans. Soft serving.

## 32.Cilantro Lime Roasted Cauliflower

Total time: 20 min

Prep time: 10 min

Cook time: 10 min

Yield: 4 servings

### Ingredients:

- 2 cups of chopped cauliflower florets
- 2 tablespoons of coconut oil, melted
- 2teaspoons of chili powder
- 1/2 teaspoon of garlic powder
- 1 medium lime
- 2 tablespoons of chopped cilantro

### Directions:

1. In a big bowl of coconut oil, combine the cauliflower. Using ground chili and garlic to scatter. Put some seasoned cauliflower in the Air Fryer basket.

2. Set the temperature to 350 degrees F and change the seven-minute timer. The cauliflower gets wet on the sides and starts to turn golden. Set it down in a bowl to eat.

3. Break the lime into quarters and spill over it with cauliflower milk. Coriander garnish.

## 33.Dinner Rolls

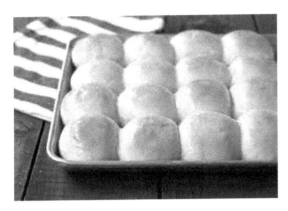

Total time: 20 min

Prep time: 10 min

Cook time: 10 min

Yield: 4 servings

### Ingredients:

- 1 cup of shredded mozzarella cheese
- 1 ounce of full-Fat: cream cheese
- 1 cup of blanched finely ground almond flour
- 1/4 cup of ground flaxseed
- ½ teaspoon of baking powder
- 1 large egg

### Directions:

1. Place the mozzarella, cream cheese, and almond flour in a large microwave-safe oven. Until flat, blend.

2. Substitute until smooth and thoroughly mixed with flaxseed, baking powder, and egg. Pulse for another 15 seconds if it gets too stiff.

3. Separate the dough into six pieces and roll the dough into balls. Put the Air Fryer balls in the basket.

4. Turn to 320° F and set the 12-minute timer.

5. Enable the rolls to cool completely before eating.

## 34.Fiery Stuffed Peppers

Preparation time: 20 minutes

Cooking time: 20 minutes

Servings: 4

### Ingredients:

- 4 medium green peppers, seeds and stems removed
- 150 g lean minced meat
- 80g grated cheddar cheese, divided
- ½ cup tomato sauce, divided
- ½ tsp. Dried mango powder
- ½ tsp. Chili powder
- ½ tsp. Turmeric powder
- 1 tsp. Worcestershire sauce
- 1 tsp. Coriander powder
- 1 onion, minced
- 1 clove garlic, minced
- 2 tsp., minced coriander leaves
- 1 tsp. Vegetable oil

### Directions:

1. Start by setting the oven to 390 degrees f for your air fryer toast.

2. Cook the peppers in salted boiling water for 3 minutes, then move them to a dish.

3. Apply the oil over medium-low heat to a small saucepan and sauté the onion and garlic for 1-2 minutes, then remove from the heat.

4. Combine all the ingredients, except half the cheese and tomato sauce, in a big bowl.

5. With the beef mixture, stuff the peppers and cover with the remaining cheese and tomato sauce.

6. Lightly oil the basket and place the 4 stuffed peppers from your air fryer toast oven.

7. Cook for 15 to 20 minutes or before you want it cooked. Enjoy!

## 35.Beef and veggies stir fry

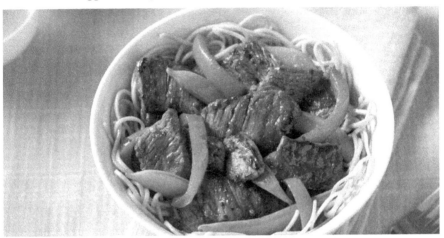

Preparation time: 45 minutes

Cooking time: 15 minutes

Servings: 4

## Ingredients:

- 450g beef sirloin, cut into strips
- 1 yellow pepper, sliced
- 1 red pepper, sliced
- 1 green pepper, sliced
- 1 broccoli, cut into florets
- 1 large red onion, sliced
- 1 large white onion, sliced
- 1 tsp. Sesame oil

- For the marinade:
- 2 tsp. Minced garlic
- 1 tbsp. Low sodium soy sauce
- ¼ cup hoisin sauce
- ¼ cup water
- 1 tsp. Sesame oil
- 1 tsp. Ground ginger

## Directions:

1. In a wide bowl, begin by whisking all the marinade ingredients. Add in the strips of beef and toss well, so all the bits are covered equally. Using cling wrap to protect it and let it stay for 30 minutes in the fridge.

2. Combine all the vegetables and the sesame oil and place the toast oven in the basket of your air fryer at 200 degrees F. For 5 minutes, cook.

3. Move the vegetables to a bowl and put the meat in your toast oven's air fryer basket.

4. Be sure that the marinade is drained. Increase the temperature and simmer for 5 minutes, to 360 degrees f. Shake the meat and cook for an additional 3 minutes, or until needed.

5. Attach the vegetables and simmer for an extra 2 minutes.

6. Serve on a steamed rice bed. Enjoy!

## 36.Air Fried Chili Beef with Toasted Cashews

Preparation time: 10 minutes

Cooking time: 25 minutes

Servings: 24

## Ingredients:

- ½ tablespoon extra-virgin olive oil or canola oil
- 450g sliced lean beef
- 2 teaspoons red curry paste
- 1 teaspoon liquid stevia, optional

- 2 tablespoons fresh lime juice
- 2 teaspoon fish sauce
- 1 cup green capsicum, diced
- ½ cup water
- 24 toasted cashews
- 1 teaspoon arrowroot starch

## Directions:

1. Set the oven to 375 degrees f for your air fryer toast.
2. Mix the beef and olive oil and fry for about 15 minutes until the inside is no longer yellow, rotating twice.
3. Apply the red curry paste and simmer for a few more minutes.
4. Mix the stevia, lime juice, fish sauce, capsicum and water in a big pot; boil for about 10 minutes.
5. To make a paste, mix cooked arrowroot with water; stir the paste into the sauce to thicken it.
6. Attach the fried cashews and remove the pan from the sun. Serve.

## 37.Beef Stir Fry W/ Red Onions & Peppers

Preparation time: 10 minutes

Cooking time: 10 minutes

Servings: 4

## Ingredients:

- 450g grass-fed flank steak, thinly sliced strips
- 1 tablespoon rice wine
- 2 teaspoons balsamic vinegar
- Pinch of sea salt
- Pinch of pepper
- 3 teaspoons extra-virgin olive oil

- 1 large yellow onion, thinly chopped
- 1/2 red bell pepper, thinly sliced
- 1/2 green bell pepper, thinly sliced
- 1 tablespoon toasted sesame seeds
- 1 teaspoon crushed red pepper flakes

## Directions:

Place meat in a bowl; stir in rice wine and vinegar, sea salt and pepper. Toss to coat well.

Set your air fryer toast oven to 375 degrees f.

Add the meat and olive and cook for about 3-5 minutes or until the meat is browned.

Heat the remaining oil on a stovetop pan and sauté onions for about 2 minutes or until caramelized; stir in pepper and cook for 2 minutes more.

Add the caramelized onions to the air fryer toast oven and stir in sesame seeds and red pepper flakes and cook for 1-2 minutes. Serve hot!

## 38.Air Fryer Toast Oven Italian Beef

Preparation time: 10 minutes

Cooking time: 1 hour 30 minutes

Servings: 8

## Ingredients:

- 1200g grass-fed chuck roast
- 6 cloves garlic
- 1 tsp. Marjoram
- 1 tsp. Basil
- 1 tsp. Oregano
- 1/2 tsp. Ground ginger
- 1 tsp. Onion powder
- 2 tsp. Garlic powder
- 1 tsp. Salt

- 1/4 cup apple cider vinegar
- 1 cup beef broth

**Directions:**

1. Cut slits in the roast with a sharp knife and then stuff with garlic cloves. In a bowl, whisk together marjoram, basil, oregano, ground ginger, onion powder, garlic powder, and salt until well blended; rub the seasoning all over the roast and place in a large air fryer toast oven pan.

2. Add vinegar and broth and lock lid; cook at 400 degrees f for 90 minutes. Take the roast out and then shred meat with a fork. Serve along with cooking juices.

### 39.Healthy Quinoa Bowl with Grilled Steak & Veggies

Preparation time: 10 minutes

Cooking time: 20 minutes

Servings: 4

**Ingredients:**

- 2 cups quinoa
- 16 ounces steak, cut into bite-size pieces
- 1 cup baby arugula
- 1 cup sweet potato slices
- 1 cup red pepper, chopped
- 1 cup scallions, chopped
- 1/2 cup toasted salted pepitas
- 2 tsp. Fresh cilantro leaves
- 2 cups microgreens
- 2 tbsp. Tomato sauce
- 2 tbsp. Extra-virgin olive oil
- Kosher salt
- Black pepper
- 1 tbsp. Fresh lime juice

**Directions:**

1. In your instant cooker, cook quinoa as needed.

2. Meanwhile, in your air-fryer toast oven, grill steak to medium rare for around 15 minutes at 350 degrees f. Grill the scallions, red pepper and sweet potatoes until tender, along with the beef.

3. Top with grilled beef, scallions, veggies, pepitas, cilantro, and microgreens. Place cooked quinoa in a bowl.

4. Combine the oil, tomato sauce, salt, and pepper in a small bowl until well blended; drizzle over the steak mixture and serve with lime juice.

## 27. Pork and Mixed Greens Salad

Preparation time: 10 minutes

Cooking time: 15 minutes

Servings: 4

**Ingredients:**

- 2 pounds pork tenderloin, slice into 1-inch slices
- 1 teaspoon dried marjoram
- 6 cups mixed salad greens
- 1 (8-ounce) package button mushrooms, sliced
- 1/3 cup low-sodium low-fat vinaigrette dressing

**Directions:**

1. Combine the olive oil and the pork slices. Toss it to coat it.

2. Sprinkle the marjoram and pepper with them and rub them onto the pork.

3. Grill the pork in batches in an air fryer until the pork on a meat thermometer hits at least 145 °f.

4. Combine the red bell pepper, salad greens, and mushrooms. Gently toss.

5. Add the slices to the salad until cooked.

6. Drizzle and toss softly with the vinaigrette. Immediately serve.

## 40.Pork Satay

Preparation time: 15 minutes

Cooking time: 14 minutes

Servings: 4

Ingredients:

- 1 (1-pound) pork tenderloin, cut into 1½-inch cubes
- ¼ cup minced onion
- 2 garlic cloves, minced
- 2 tablespoons freshly squeezed lime juice, coconut milk, curry powder
- 2 tablespoons unsalted peanut butter

Directions:

1. Combine the ham, ginger, garlic, jalapeño, coconut milk, lime juice, peanut butter, and curry powder with the mixture. Place it aside at room temperature for 10 minutes.

2. From the marinade, take the pork out. Marinade Reserve.

3. Onto approximately 8 bamboo skewers, string the pork. With the reserved marinade, grill and clean once, before the pork on a meat thermometer hits at least 145 °f. Discard every marinade that exists. Immediately serve.

## 41.Pork Burgers with Red Cabbage Salad

Preparation time: 20 minutes

Cooking time: 9 minutes

Servings: 4

Ingredients:

- ½ cup greek yogurt
- 2 tablespoons low-sodium mustard, paprika
- 1 tablespoon lemon juice
- ¼ cup red cabbage, carrots
- 1-pound lean ground pork

Directions:

1. Combine 1 tablespoon of mustard, lemon juice, cabbage, and carrots with the yogurt; blend and cool.

2. Combine the bacon, 1 tablespoon of mustard left, and the paprika. Mold into eight little patties.

3. Insert the sliders into the basket of the air fryer. Grill with a meat thermometer until the sliders register 165 ° f as checked.

4. By putting some of the lettuce greens on a bun bottom, arrange the burgers. Cover it with a slice of onion, tacos, and a combination of cabbage. Attach the top of the bun and quickly serve.

## 42.Crispy Mustard Pork Tenderloin

Preparation time: 10 minutes

Cooking time: 12 to 16 minutes

Servings: 4

### Ingredients:

- 3 tablespoons low-sodium grainy mustard
- ¼ teaspoon dry mustard powder
- 1 (1-pound) pork tenderloin
- ¼ cup ground walnuts
- 2 tablespoons cornstarch

### Directions:

26. Stir together the mustard, olive oil, and mustard powder. Spread this mixture over the pork.

27. On a plate, mix the bread crumbs, walnuts, and cornstarch. Dip the mustard-coated pork into the crumb mixture to coat.

28. Air-fry the pork until it registers at least 145°f on a meat thermometer. Slice to serve.

## 43.Apple Pork Tenderloin

Preparation time: 10 minutes

Cooking time: 14 to 19 minutes

Servings: 4

### Ingredients:

- 1 (1-pound) pork tenderloin, cut into 4 pieces
- 1 tablespoon apple butter
- 2 granny smith apples or Jonagold apples, sliced
- ½ teaspoon dried marjoram
- 1/3 cup apple juice

### Directions:

1. Rub the apple butter and olive oil with each slice of pork.
2. Mix together the bacon, apples, 3 celery, 1 marjoram, 1 cabbage, and apple juice.
3. Place the bowl in the fryer and roast until the pork on a meat thermometer hits at least 145 ° f, and the apples and vegetables are tender. During cooking, stir once. Immediately serve.

## 44.Espresso-Grilled Pork Tenderloin

Preparation time: 15 minutes

Cooking time: 9 to 11 minutes

Servings: 4

### Ingredients:

- 2 teaspoons espresso powder
- 1 teaspoon ground paprika
- ½ teaspoon dried marjoram
- 1 tablespoon honey, lemon juice, brown sugar
- 1 (1-pound) pork tenderloin

### Directions:

Combine the brown sugar, marjoram, paprika, and espresso powder.

Stir in the olive oil, lemon juice and honey until well combined.

Spread the honey mixture over the pork and let it rest at room temperature for 10 minutes.

In the air fryer basket, roast the tenderloin until the pork reports at least 145°f on a meat thermometer. To cook, slice the beef.

## 45.Garlic Lamb Chops with Thyme

Preparation time: 10 minutes

Cooking time: 30 minutes

Servings: 4

## Ingredients:

- 4 lamb chops
- 1 garlic clove, peeled
- 1 tbsp. plus
- 2 tsp. olive oil
- ½ tbsp. oregano
- ½ tbsp. thyme
- ½ tsp. salt
- ¼ tsp. black pepper

## Directions:

1. Preheat the fryer to 390 f for air. Coat the clove of garlic with 1 tsp. Olive oil and put for 10 minutes in the air fryer. Meanwhile, with the remaining olive oil, combine the herbs and seasonings.

2. Squeeze the hot roasted garlic clove into the herb mixture using a towel or a mitten, and stir to blend. Coat the mixture well with the lamb chops, and put them in the air fryer. For 8 to 12 minutes, cook.

3.

## 46.Lamb Meatloaf

Preparation time: 15 minutes

Cooking time: 40 minutes

Servings: 4

**Ingredients:**

- 2 lb. Lamb, ground
- 4 scallions; chopped
- 1 egg
- A drizzle of olive oil
- 2 tbsp. Tomato sauce
- 2 tbsp. Parsley; chopped
- 2 tbsp. Cilantro; chopped
- ¼ tsp. Cinnamon powder
- 1 tsp. Coriander, ground
- 1 tsp. Lemon juice
- ½ tsp. Hot paprika
- 1 tsp. Cumin, ground
- A pinch of salt and black pepper

**Directions:**

1. Combine the lamb in a bowl with the rest of the ingredients, except for the oil, and mix very well.
2. Grease a loaf pan that suits the oil in the air fryer, add the lamb mix and mold the meatloaf
3. Place the pan in an air fryer and cook for 35 minutes at 380 °f. Slicing and serving

4.

## 47.Lamb Chops and Mint Sauce

Preparation time: 10 minutes

Cooking time: 29 minutes

Servings: 4

### Ingredients:

- 8 lamb chops
- 1 cup mint; chopped
- 1 garlic clove; minced
- 2 tbsp. Olive oil
- Juice of 1 lemon
- A pinch of salt and black pepper

### Directions:

1. Combine all the ingredients in a blender, except the lamb, and pulse well.

2. Rub lamb chops with the mint sauce, place them in your air fryer's basket and cook at 400°f for 12 minutes on each side

3. Divide and serve everything between plates.

4.

## 48.Rosemary Roasted Lamb Cutlets

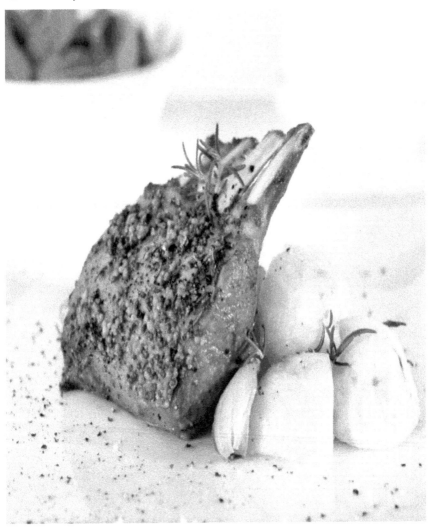

Preparation time: 15 minutes

Cooking time: 35 minutes

Servings: 4

**Ingredients:**

- 8 lamb cutlets

- 2 garlic cloves; minced
- 2 tbsp. Rosemary; chopped
- 2 tbsp. Olive oil
- A pinch of salt and black pepper
- A pinch of cayenne pepper

**Directions:**

1. Take a bowl and mix the rest of the ingredients with the lamb: rub well.
2. Place the lamb in the fryer's basket and cook for 30 minutes at 380°f, flipping halfway. Divide between plates and serve the cutlets

## 49.Seasoned Lamb

Preparation time: 15 minutes

Cooking time: 40 minutes

Servings: 4

**Ingredients:**

- 1 lb. Lamb leg; boneless and sliced
- ½ cup walnuts; chopped
- 2 garlic cloves; minced
- 1 tbsp. Parsley; chopped
- 1 tbsp. Rosemary; chopped
- 2 tbsp. Olive oil
- ¼ tsp. Red pepper flakes
- ½ tsp. Mustard seeds
- ½ tsp. Italian seasoning
- A pinch of salt and black pepper

**Directions:**

1. Take a bowl and combine the lamb with all the ingredients: rub well except the walnuts and parsley, place the slices in the basket of your air fryer and cook for 35 minutes at 370 ° F, flipping the meat halfway.

2. Spread the parsley and walnuts on top and serve with a side salad. Split between dishes.

## 50.Herbed Lamb

Preparation time: 15 minutes

Cooking time: 40 minutes

Servings: 4

**Ingredients:**

- 8 lamb cutlets
- ¼ cup mustard
- 2 garlic cloves; minced
- 1 tbsp. Oregano; chopped
- 1 tbsp. Mint chopped.
- 1 tbsp. Chives; chopped
- 1 tbsp. Basil; chopped
- A drizzle of olive oil
- A pinch of salt and black pepper

**Directions:**

1. Take a bowl and mix the rest of the ingredients with the lamb: rub well.
2. Place the cutlets in the basket of your air fryer and cook on each side at 380°f for 15 minutes.
3. Divide and serve with a side salad between dishes.

## 51.Rack of Lamb

Preparation time: 5 minutes

Cooking time: 10 minutes

Servings: 2 to 4

**Ingredients:**

- 1 rack of lamb
- 2 tbsp. Of dried rosemary

- 1 tbsp. Of dried thyme
- 2 tsp. Of minced garlic
- Salt
- Pepper
- 4 tbsp. Of olive oil

## Directions:

1. Start by combining the herbs, mixing the rosemary, thyme, garlic, salt, pepper, and olive oil in a small bowl and combine well.

2. Rub the mixture all over the lamb, then. Place the lamb rack inside the air fryer. Set the temperature for about 10 minutes, to 360f.

3. After 10 minutes, use the method above to calculate the internal temperature of the lamb rack. It will be 145 f if you want an uncommon one.

4. That will be 160 f if you want a medium. If you'd like to do well, it would be 170 f. Remove the bowls, then serve.

## 52.Lamb Sirloin Steak

Preparation time: 40 minutes

Cooking time: 15 minutes

Servings: 2 to 4

## Ingredients:

- ½ onions
- 4 slices of ginger
- 5 cloves of garlic
- 1 tsp. of garam masala
- 1 tsp. Of ground fennel
- 1 tsp. Of ground cinnamon
- ½ tsp. Of ground cardamom
- 1 tsp. Of cayenne
- 1 tsp. Of salt

- 1 lb. Of boneless lamb sirloin steaks

## Directions:

1. Add all the ingredients to a blender bowl, except the lamb chops.

2. Pulse and blend until the onion and all ingredients are finely minced: blend for around 3 to 4 minutes.

3. Place the chops of the lamb into a side dish. To allow the marinade to penetrate better, use a knife to slice the meat and fat.

4. Toss well the mixed spice paste and combine well. Enable the mixture to rest for 30 minutes or in the refrigerator for up to 24 hours.

5. For about 15 minutes, allow your air fryer to 330 f and place the lamb steaks in the air fryer basket in a single layer and cook, flipping halfway through.

6. Ensure that the meat has reached an inner temperature of 150f for medium-well, using a meat thermometer, and serve.

## 53.Beef Pork Meatballs

Preparation time: 10 minutes

Cooking time: 20 minutes

Servings: 6

## Ingredients:

- 1 lb. Ground beef
- 1 lb. Ground pork
- 1/2 cup Italian breadcrumbs
- 1/3 cup milk
- 1/4 cup onion, diced
- 1/2 teaspoon garlic powder
- 1 teaspoon Italian seasoning
- 1 egg
- 1/4 cup parsley chopped
- 1/4 cup shredded parmesan

- Salt and pepper to taste

## Directions:

1. In a bowl, carefully mix the beef with all the other meatball ingredients.

2. Create tiny meatballs out of this combination, then put them in the basket of the air fryer.

3. Click the Air Fry Oven control button and switch the knob to pick the bake mode.

4. To set the cooking time to 20 minutes, click the time button and change the dial once again.

5. Now press the temp button to set the temperature at 400 degrees f and rotate the dial.

6. When preheated, put the basket of meatballs in the oven and close the lid.

7. When baked, turn the meatballs halfway through and then start cooking.

8. Serve it hot.

## 54. Beef Noodle Casserole

Preparation time: 10 minutes

Cooking time: 35 minutes

Servings: 6

## Ingredients:

- 2 tablespoons olive oil
- 1 medium onion, chopped
- ½ lb. Ground beef
- 4 fresh mushrooms, sliced
- 1 cup pasta noodles, cooked
- 2 cups marinara sauce
- 1 teaspoon butter
- 4 teaspoons flour

- 1 cup milk
- 1 egg, beaten
- 1 cup cheddar cheese, grated

Directions:

29. Put a wok on moderate heat and add oil to heat.

30. Toss in onion and sauté until soft.

31. Stir in mushrooms and beef, then cook until meat is brown.

32. Add marinara sauce and cook it to a simmer.

33. Stir in pasta then spread this mixture in a casserole dish.

34. Prepare the sauce by melting butter in a saucepan over moderate heat.

35. Stir in flour and whisk well, pour in the milk.

36. Mix well and whisk ¼ cup sauce with egg, then return it to the saucepan.

37. Stir, cook for 1 minute, then pour this sauce over the beef.

38. Drizzle cheese over the beef casserole.

39. Press the "power button" of the air fry oven and turn the dial to select the "bake" mode.

40. Press the time button and again turn the dial to set the cooking time to 30 minutes.

41. Now push the temp button and rotate the dial to set the temperature at 350 degrees f.

42. Once preheated, place the casserole dish in the oven and close its lid.

43. Serve warm.

## 55.Saucy Beef Bake

Preparation time: 10 minutes

Cooking time: 36 minutes

Servings: 6

### Ingredients:

- 2 tablespoons olive oil
- 1 large onion, diced

- 2 lbs. Ground beef
- 2 teaspoons salt
- 6 cloves garlic, chopped
- 1/2 cup red wine
- 6 cloves garlic, chopped
- 3 teaspoons ground cinnamon
- 2 teaspoons ground cumin
- 2 teaspoons dried oregano
- 1 teaspoon black pepper
- 1 can 28 oz. Crushed tomatoes
- 1 tablespoon tomato paste

**Directions:**

1. In a bowl, carefully mix the beef with all the other meatball ingredients.
2. Create tiny meatballs out of this combination, then put them in the basket of the air fryer.
3. Click the Air Fry Oven control button and switch the knob to pick the bake mode.
4. To set the cooking time to 20 minutes, click the time button and change the dial once again.
5. Now press the temp button to set the temperature at 400 degrees f and rotate the dial.
6. When preheated, put the basket of meatballs in the oven and close the lid.
7. When baked, turn the meatballs halfway through and then start cooking.
8. Serve it hot.

### 56.Beets and Arugula Salad

Total time: 20 min

Prep time: 10 min

Cook time: 10 min

Yield: 4 servings

**Ingredients:**

- 1 and ½ pounds of beets, peeled and quartered
- A drizzle of olive oil
- 2 teaspoons of orange zest, grated
- 2 tablespoons of cider vinegar
- ½ cup of orange juice
- 2 tablespoons of brown sugar
- 2 scallions, chopped
- 2 teaspoons of mustard
- 2 cups of arugula

**Directions:**

1. Rub the beets with the orange juice and oil, put them in your Air Fryer, and cook at 350 °F for 10 minutes.
2. Move the beet quarters to a bowl, add the scallions, arugula zest, and orange and blend.
3. In a separate dish, blend the sugar with the mustard and vinegar, blend properly, add the lettuce, whisk and eat.

## 57. Beet Tomato and Goat Cheese Mix

Total time: 45 min

Prep time: 20 min

Cook time: 25 min

Yield: 8 servings

**Ingredients:**

- 8 small beets, trimmed, peeled, and halved
- 1 red onion, sliced
- 4 ounces of goat cheese, crumbled
- 1 tablespoon of balsamic vinegar

- Salt and black pepper to the taste
- 2 tablespoons of sugar
- 1-pint mixed cherry tomatoes halved
- 2 ounces of pecans
- 2 tablespoons of olive oil

Directions:

1. Connect the beets to the Air Fryer, season with salt and pepper, cook for 14 minutes at 350 °F and move to a salad bowl.
2. Attach the carrot, pecans, and cherry tomatoes, and toss.
3. Mix the vinegar with the sugar and oil in another dish, stir well until the sugar dissolves, and add to the salad.
4. Add goat cheese as well, toss, and eat.

## 58.Broccoli Salad

Total time: 20 min

Prep time: 10 min

Cook time: 10 min

Yield: 8 servings

Ingredients:

- 1 broccoli head, florets separated
- 1 tablespoon of peanut oil
- 6 garlic cloves, minced
- 1 tablespoon of Chinese rice wine vinegar
- Salt and black pepper to the taste

Directions:

1. In a cup, mix broccoli with salt, pepper and half the oil, shake, switch to your Air Fryer, and cook at 350 °F for 8 minutes, shaking halfway through the fryer.
2. Transfer the broccoli and the leftover peanut oil, garlic and rice vinegar into a salad bowl, blend well and eat very nicely.

## 59.Brussels Sprouts and Tomatoes Mix

Total time: 15 min

Prep time: 5 min

Cook time: 10 min

Yield: 4 servings

Ingredients:

- 1-pound of Brussels sprouts, trimmed
- Salt and black pepper to the taste
- 6 cherry tomatoes, halved
- ¼ cup of green onions, chopped
- 1 tablespoon of olive oil

Directions:

1. Season Brussels with salt and pepper sprouts, put in your fryer and cook at 350 degrees F for 10 minutes.
2. Add salt, pepper, cherry tomatoes, olive oil, and green onions, blend well and eat. Put them in a cup.

## 60.Brussels Sprouts and Butter Sauce

Total time: 15 min

Prep time: 5 min

Cook time: 10 min

Yield: 4 servings

Ingredients:

- 1-pound of Brussels sprouts, trimmed
- Salt and black pepper to the taste
- ½ cup of bacon, cooked and chopped
- 1 tablespoon of mustard
- 1 tablespoon of butter
- 2 tablespoons dill, finely chopped

**Directions:**

1. In the Air Fryer, put the Brussels sprouts and cook them at 350 °F for 10 minutes.

2. Heat a skillet with the butter over medium-high heat, add the bacon, mustard, and dill and whisk well.

3. In Brussels, split the sprouts between bowls, drizzle the butter sauce all over, and eat.

## 61.Cheesy Brussels sprouts

Total time: 18 min

Prep time: 5 min

Cook time: 10 min

Yield: 4 servings

### Ingredients:

- 1-pound of Brussels sprouts washed

- Juice of 1 lemon

- Salt and black pepper to the taste

- 2 tablespoons of butter

- 3 tablespoons of parmesan, grated

### Directions:

1. Put the sprouts in the Brussels Air Fryer, cook them at 350 degrees F for 8 minutes, and position them on a tray.

2. Heat the butter in a skillet over medium heat, add the lemon juice, salt and pepper, stir well and add the Brussels sprouts.

3. Before the parmesan melts, add the parmesan, toss and serve.

## 62.Spicy Cabbage

Total time: 18 min

Prep time: 5 min

Cook time: 10 min

Yield: 4 servings

Ingredients:

- 1 cabbage, cut into 8 wedges
- 1 tablespoon of sesame seed oil
- 1 carrot, grated
- ¼ cup of apple cider vinegar
- ¼ cups of apple juice
- ½ teaspoon of cayenne pepper
- 1 teaspoon of red pepper flakes, crushed

Directions:

1. Combine cabbage with oil, carrot, vinegar, apple juice, cayenne, and pepper flakes, shake, put in preheated Air Fryer, and cook for 8 minutes at 350° F in a pan that suits your Air Fryer.

2. Divide and serve cabbage mixture on bowls.

### 63.Sweet Baby Carrots Dish

Total time: 20 min

Prep time: 5 min

Cook time: 15 min

Yield: 4 servings

Ingredients:

- 2 cups of baby carrots
- A pinch of salt and black pepper
- 1 tablespoon of brown sugar
- ½ tablespoon of butter, melted

Directions:

1. In a dish that fits your Air Fryer blend, add baby carrots with butter, salt, pepper and sugar, place in your Air Fryer, and cook at 350 °F for 10 minutes.

2. Divide and feed between bowls.

## 64.Collard Greens Mix

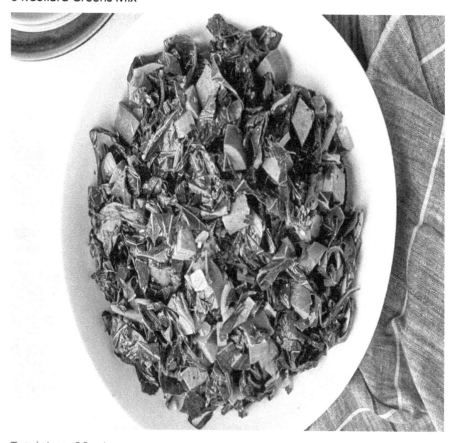

Total time: 20 min

Prep time: 5 min

Cook time: 15 min

Yield: 4 servings

**Ingredients:**

- 1 bunch of collard greens, trimmed
- 2 tablespoons of olive oil
- 2 tablespoons of tomato puree
- 1 yellow onion, chopped
- 3 garlic cloves, minced
- Salt and black pepper to the taste

- 1 tablespoon of balsamic vinegar
- 1 teaspoon of sugar

**Directions:**

1. In a bowl that matches your Air Fryer, mix the oil, garlic, vinegar, onion, and tomato puree and whisk.
2. Add the collard greens, salt, pepper and shake with the butter, stir in the Air Fryer and roast at 320 degrees F for 10 minutes.
3. Divide the collard greens into bowls and serve

## 65.Collard Greens and Turkey Wings

Total time: 30 min

Prep time: 10 min

Cook time: 25 min

Yield: 2 servings

**Ingredients:**

- 1 sweet onion, chopped
- 2 smoked turkey wings
- 2 tablespoons of olive oil
- 3 garlic cloves, minced
- 2 and ½ pounds of collard greens, chopped
- Salt and black pepper to the taste
- 2 tablespoons of apple cider vinegar
- 1 tablespoon of brown sugar
- ½ teaspoon of crushed red pepper

**Directions:**

1. Heat up a medium-hot saucepan that suits the grease of your Air Fryer, add the onions, stir and cook for 2 minutes.
2. Connect the garlic, the onions, the mustard, the salt, the pepper, the crushed red pepper, the cinnamon and the smoked turkey, add the preheated Air Fryer and cook at 350 degrees F for 15 minutes.

## 66.Herbed Eggplant and Zucchini Mix

Total time: 18 min

Prep time: 5 min

Cook time: 10 min

Yield: 4 servings

### Ingredients:

- 1 eggplant, roughly cubed
- 3 zucchinis, roughly cubed
- 2 tablespoons of lemon juice
- Salt and black pepper to the taste
- 1 teaspoon of thyme, dried
- 1 teaspoon of oregano, dried
- 3 tablespoons of olive oil

### Directions:

1. Place the eggplant in the bowl of the Air Fryer, add the zucchini, lemon juice, salt, pepper, thyme, oregano and olive oil, blend and place in the Air Fryer and cook for 8 minutes at 360 degrees F.
2. Divide into bowls and instantly serve.

## 67.Flavored Fennel

Total time: 18 min

Prep time: 5 min

Cook time: 10 min

Yield: 4 servings

### Ingredients:

- 2 fennel bulbs, cut into quarters
- 3 tablespoons of olive oil
- Salt and black pepper to the taste
- 1 garlic clove, minced

- 1 red chili pepper, chopped
- ¾ cup of veggie stock
- Juice from ½ lemon
- ¼ cup of white wine
- ¼ cup of parmesan, grated

## Directions:

1. Heat a medium-hot saucepan that fits the oil with your Air Fryer, add the garlic and chili pepper, stir and cook for 2 minutes.

2. Add the fennel, salt, pepper, stock, vinegar, lemon juice and parmesan, cover with a swirl, throw in the Air Fryer and cook at 350 °F for 6 minutes.

3. Divide them into plates.

### 68.Okra and Corn Salad

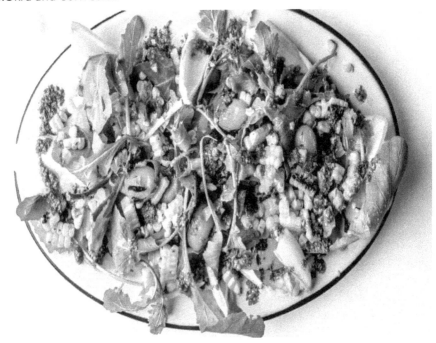

Total time: 20 min

Prep time: 5 min

Cook time: 15 min

Yield: 4 servings

**Ingredients:**

- 3 green bell peppers, chopped
- 2 tablespoons of olive oil
- 1 teaspoon of sugar
- 1-pound of okra, trimmed
- 6 scallions, chopped
- Salt and black pepper to the taste
- 28 ounces of canned tomatoes, chopped
- 1 cup of corn

**Directions:**

1. Heat a pan over medium-high heat that suits the oil with your Air Fryer, add bell peppers and scallions, blend and cook for 5 minutes.
2. Connect the okra, salt, pepper, sugar, tomatoes, and maize, stir, put in the Air Fryer and cook at 360 degrees F for 7 minutes.
3. Break the mixture of okra into plates and serve until wet.

## 69.Air Fried Leeks

Total time: 18 min

Prep time: 5 min

Cook time: 10 min

Yield: 4 servings

**Ingredients:**

- 4 leeks, washed, ends cut off and halved
- Salt and black pepper to the taste
- 1 tablespoon of butter, melted
- 1 tablespoon of lemon juice

**Directions:**

1. Rub the leeks with the melted butter, season with salt and pepper, add to the Air Fryer and cook at 350 degrees F for 7 minutes.

2. Set the lemon juice on a pan, drizzle it all over and eat.

## 70.Crispy Potatoes and Parsley

Total time: 20 min

Prep time: 5 min

Cook time: 15 min

Yield: 4 servings

### Ingredients:

- 1-pound of gold potatoes, cut into wedges
- Salt and black pepper to the taste
- 2 tablespoons of olive
- Juice from ½ lemon
- ¼ cup of parsley leaves, chopped

Directions:

1. Rub the potatoes with salt, pepper, lemon juice and olive oil, add them to the Air Fryer and cook at 350 degrees F for 10 minutes.

2. Sprinkle on top of the parsley, break into bowls and eat.

## 71.Indian Turnips Salad

Total time: 22 min

Prep time: 7 min

Cook time: 15 min

Yield: 4 servings

### Ingredients:

- 20 ounces of turnips, peeled and chopped
- 1 teaspoon of garlic, minced
- 1 teaspoon of ginger, grated
- 2 yellow onions, chopped

- 2 tomatoes, chopped
- 1 teaspoon of cumin, ground
- 1 teaspoon of coriander, ground
- 2 green chilies, chopped
- ½ teaspoon of turmeric powder
- 2 tablespoons of butter
- Salt and black pepper to the taste
- A handful of coriander leaves, chopped

**Directions:**

1. In a saucepan that fits your Air Fryer, heats the butter, melt it, add the green chilies, garlic, and ginger, stir and cook for 1 minute.
2. Add the onions, salt, pepper, tomatoes, turmeric, cumin, cilantro and turnips, stir, put in the Air Fryer and cook at 350 degrees F. for 10 minutes.
3. Break into cups, sprinkle with fresh coriander on top and serve.

## 72.Simple Stuffed Tomatoes

Total time: 25 min

Prep time: 10 min

Cook time: 15 min

Yield: 6 servings

**Ingredients:**

- 4 tomatoes, tops cut off and pulp scooped and chopped
- Salt and black pepper to the taste
- 1 yellow onion, chopped
- 1 tablespoon of butter
- 2 tablespoons of celery, chopped
- ½ cup of mushrooms, chopped
- 1 tablespoon of bread crumbs
- 1 cup of cottage cheese

- ¼ teaspoon of caraway seeds
- 1 tablespoon of parsley, chopped

**Directions:**

1. Heat a saucepan with the butter over medium heat, melt, add the onion and celery, stir and simmer for 3 minutes.
2. Link the mushrooms and tomato pulp and then stir and boil for 1 minute.
3. Add salt, pepper, crumbled bread, cheese, parsley, caraway seeds, stir, cook for another 4 minutes, and heat up.
4. With this blend, stuff the tomatoes, place them in the Air Fryer, and cook at 350 °F for 8 minutes.
5. Divide the stewed tomatoes into bowls and serve.

## 73.Indian Potatoes

Total time: 22 min

Prep time: 7 min

Cook time: 15 min

Yield: 4 servings

**Ingredients:**

- 1 tablespoon of coriander seeds
- 1 tablespoon of cumin seeds
- Salt and black pepper to the taste
- ½ teaspoon of turmeric powder
- ½ teaspoon of red chili powder
- 1 teaspoon of pomegranate powder
- 1 tablespoon of pickled mango, chopped
- 2 teaspoons of fenugreek, dried
- 5 potatoes, boiled, peeled, and cubed
- 2 tablespoons of olive oil

**Directions:**

1. Over medium pressure, heat a saucepan that suits the oil of your Air Fryer, add the coriander and cumin seeds, stir and simmer for 2 minutes.

2. Add cinnamon, pepper, turmeric, chili powder, mango, fenugreek, pomegranate powder and potatoes, blend, add Air Fryer and simmer at 360 °F for 10 minutes.

3. Divide and serve sweetly between bowls.

## 74. Broccoli and Tomatoes Air Fried Stew

Total time: 30 min

Prep time: 10 min

Cook time: 25 min

Yield: 2 servings

### Ingredients:

- 1 broccoli head, florets separated
- 2 teaspoons of coriander seeds
- 1 tablespoon of olive oil
- 1 yellow onion, chopped
- Salt and black pepper to the taste
- A pinch of red pepper, crushed
- 1 small ginger piece, chopped
- 1 garlic clove, minced
- 28 ounces of canned tomatoes, pureed

### Directions:

1. Heat a medium-hot pan that matches the oil with your Air Fryer, add the onions, salt, pepper, and red pepper, combine and cook for seven minutes.

2. Add the ginger, garlic, cilantro, tomatoes and broccoli, stir, add to the Air Fryer and cook at 360 degrees F for 12 minutes.

3. Break and serve in pots.

## 75. Collard Greens and Bacon

Total time: 22 min

Prep time: 7 min

Cook time: 15 min

Yield: 4 servings

## Ingredients:

- 1-pound collard greens
- 3 bacon strips, chopped
- ¼ cup cherry tomatoes halved
- 1 tablespoon of apple cider vinegar
- 2 tablespoons of chicken stock
- Salt and black pepper to the taste

Directions:

1. Heat a medium-pressure saucepan, add the bacon, stir and cook for 1-2 minutes.

2. Add the tomatoes, collard greens, vinegar, stock, salt and pepper, blend, add to the Air Fryer and cook at 320 degrees F for 10 minutes.

3. Divide and feed between bowls.

## 76.Sesame Mustard Greens

Total time: 22 min

Prep time: 7 min

Cook time: 15 min

Yield: 4 servings

## Ingredients:

- 2 garlic cloves, minced
- 1-pound of mustard greens, torn
- 1 tablespoon of olive oil
- ½ cup yellow onion, sliced
- Salt and black pepper to the taste

- 3 tablespoons of veggie stock
- ¼ teaspoon of dark sesame oil

Directions:

1. Heat a medium-hot saucepan that suits the grease of your Air Fryer, add the onions, blend and brown for 5 minutes.
2. Add the garlic, stock, onions, salt, and pepper, stir, add to the Air Fryer, and cook at 350 degrees F for 6 minutes.
3. Tie the sesame oil together, swirl to coat, break and serve in cups.

## 77.Radish Hash

Total time: 18 min

Prep time: 5 min

Cook time: 10 min

Yield: 4 servings

Ingredients:

- ½ teaspoon of onion powder
- 1-pound radishes, sliced
- ½ teaspoon of garlic powder
- Salt and black pepper to the taste
- 4 eggs
- 1/3 cup of parmesan, grated

Directions:

1. In a bowl of salt, pepper, onion and garlic powder, eggs, and parmesan cheese, combine the radishes, then whisk well.
2. Shift the radishes into a fridge-friendly saucepan and simmer at 350° F for 7 minutes.
3. Divide the hash into bowls and serve.

## 78.Cod Pie with Palmit
Preparation Time: 15 Minutes

Cooking Time: 30 Minutes

Servings: 4-6

**Ingredients:**

- 2 ¼ lb cod
- 4 ½ lb of natural heart previously grated and cooked
- 12 eggs
- 1 ½ cup olive oil
- 7 oz. of olives
- Tomato Chopped garlic, paprika and sliced onion
- Green seasoning

**Directions:**

1. In a frying pan, cook the cod and, after cooking, destroy it.

2. Drain the heart of the palm well on the reservation.

3. Along with tomatoes, garlic, paprika, ginger, green seasoning and half of the pitted olives, sauté the cod and palm hearts in olive oil for 20 minutes.

4. Pour 6 eggs into the sample and stir for 5 minutes.

5. Grease the olive oil trays and place the mixture into them.

6. Beat the rest of the eggs and spill over the top evenly.

7. Add tomatoes and olives to garnish.

8. Bake for 40 minutes in the air-fryer at 3800F.

### 79.Simple and Yummy Cod
Preparation Time: 10 Minutes

Cooking Time: 15 Minutes

Servings: 4-6

**Ingredients:**

- 2 ¼ lb of desalted cod
- 1 ½ lb of boiled and squeezed potatoes
- 1 can of sour cream
- 2 large onions, sliced

- 1 pot of pitted olive
- ½ cup of olive oil
- Butter for greasing

Directions:

1. In the oil, marinate the onions until they wilt.

2. Give the cod a further 5 minutes to sauté.

3. Add the sour cream and potato and stir for another 5 minutes.

4. Turn the heat off and add some more oil.

5. Place the cod in a refractory greased butter and pass the margarine over it again to render it golden.

6. Bake at 4000F for about 20 minutes or until golden brown in an air fryer.

7. It's fast and delicious to serve with rice.

## 80.Roasted Tilapia Fillet
Preparation Time: 10 Minutes

Cooking Time: 15 Minutes

Servings: 4-6

Ingredients:

- 2 ¼ lb tilapia fillet
- ½ lemon juice
- 4 sliced tomatoes
- 4 sliced onions
- ½ cup chopped black olives
- 1 pound of boiled potatoes
- 1 tbsp. butter ½ cup sour cream tea
- ½ lb grated mozzarella Olive oil Salt

Directions:

1. With lemon and salt, season the fillets.

2. Place a sheet of onions and tomatoes on an ovenproof tray. On top of the layers, position the fillets.

3. Marinade with another layer of tomato and onion, then the olives and drizzle with the olive oil.

4. Bake in an air-fryer for 15 minutes at 3600F.

5. Squeeze the potatoes in another bowl.

6. Melt the butter in a saucepan. Put the cream with both the potatoes.

7. Place this puree on top of the fillets, then place the mozzarella on top of them.

8. Bake for another 5 minutes in an air fryer at 3600F and serve.

### 81. Cod 7-Mares
Preparation Time: 10 Minutes

Cooking Time: 15 Minutes

Servings: 4-6

**Ingredients:**

- 1 lb cod in French fries
- 4 large potatoes, peeled and diced
- 1 can of cream without serum
- 1 cup of coffee with coconut milk
- 3 ½ oz. of mozzarella cheese in strips
- 3 ½ oz. cheese in pieces
- 100 g3 ½ oz. grated Parmesan cheese
- Aromatic herbs and salt to taste.
- 1 tbsp. of curry
- Salt to taste

**Directions:**

1. Cook and set aside the peeled and diced potatoes.

2. Remove the salt from the cod (leave it overnight in the water and at least change the water

3 times to have the salt erased). 3. Place the potatoes in a glass jar and cook in the microwave for 5 minutes. Set aside.

4. The cream, coconut milk, curry, mozzarella cheese, and herbs are mixed in a bowl. Mounting Up

5. Top a layer of boiled potatoes on a pan, put the cod fries on top, and pour the sauce on top.

6. Season to taste with salt.

7. Sprinkle with Parmesan cheese and cook in an air fryer at 3600F for 7 minutes.

8. Toss the chives over the top when done, and immediately serve.

## 82.Roasted Hake with Coconut Milk
Preparation Time: 10 Minutes

Cooking Time: 30 Minutes

Servings: 2

### Ingredients:

- 2 ¼ lb hake fillet
- ½ lb sliced mozzarella
- 1 can of sour cream
- 1 bottle of coconut milk
- 1 onion
- 1 tomato
- Salt and black pepper to taste.
- Lemon juice

### Directions:

1. With salt, pepper and lemon, season the fillets.

2. Let them stand for ten minutes.

3. Arrange the fillets and put each one in the center of the mozzarella slices and roll it up like a fillet.

4. The fillets were rolled up after all.

5. Just get a tray.

6. Place on top of the tomato and onion slices (sliced).

7. Attach the sour cream and coconut milk mixture to the top.

8. Bake for 20 minutes inside an air-fryer at 4000, coated with aluminum foil.

9. Then, to finish baking, remove it.

## 83.Air fryer Catfish

Preparation Time: 15 Minutes

Cooking Time: 1 Hour

Servings: 2-4

### Ingredients:

- 3 pounds sliced dogfish
- 1 pound boiled and sliced potatoes
- 1 package of onion cream
- 3 tomatoes cut into slices
- 3 bell peppers cut into slices
- 3 onions cut into slices
- Olive oil
- 2 garlic cloves, crushed
- Salt to taste
- 1 lemon juice

### Directions:

1. With garlic, salt and ginger, season the fish slices and set them aside.

2. Place the potatoes on a baking sheet to get the slices and drizzle with plenty of oil, forming a kind of bed.

3. On the potatoes, spread half of the onion cream.

4. Lay on top of the slices.

5. Place on top of the tomato, bell pepper and onion, spread well and cover the slices. Drizzle with olive oil again, and then pour on top of the rest of the onion cream.

6. Heat the air fryer at 3600F for about 15 minutes and then bake for 1 hour.

## 84.Squid to the Milanese

Preparation Time: 5 Minutes

Cooking Time: 15 Minutes

Servings: 4-6

### Ingredients:

- 2 ¼ lb clean squid
- Salt, pepper and oregano to taste.
- 3 beaten eggs
- 1 cup of wheat flour
- 1 cup breadcrumbs
- 1 cup chopped green chives

### Directions:

1. Season the squid with salt, pepper and oregano, after washing and cutting into rings.

2. Put the squid over the beaten eggs, then mix the breadcrumbs with the wheat flour.

3. Fry for 10 minutes in the air-fryer at 4000F. 4. Green onions are sprinkled.

## 85.Portugal Codfish with Cream

Preparation Time: 10 Minutes

Cooking Time: 15 Minutes

Servings: 2-4

### Ingredients:

- 2 ¼ lbs of cod
- 1 chopped onion
- 2 cloves of garlic
- 4 medium potatoes
- 1 leek stalk (Portugal leek)

- 2 cups of cream
- 1 egg Parmesan
- Coriander (optional)
- Olive oil
- Black olives

**Directions:**

1. Soak the cod in water for approximately 24 hours until the salt is to your taste.

2. Put the oil and brown the garlic, the onion and the leek in a frying pan, then place the cod and let it brown.

3. Take the diced potatoes and cook them separately.

4. Then, with the golden cod, bring the potatoes together. Then put the cilantro along with the cream or sour cream to your liking. Integrate everything.

5. Spread a little Parmesan on top, beat 1 whole egg and sprinkle the cod and marinade with black olives.

6. Place it at 3600F for 30 minutes in an air fryer or until it turns into a crispy cone.

7. Serve with a lovely salad of lettuce, nothing more.

## 86.Roasted Salmon with Provencal
Preparation Time: 10 Minutes

Cooking Time: 20 Minutes

Servings: 2

**Ingredients:**

- 4 slices of fresh salmon basil thyme
- Rosemary oregano salt and pepper olive oil
- 4 tablespoons of butter
- ½ lemon juice

**Directions:**

1. On a hot plate, place the salmon slices and sprinkle with the 4 herbs.

2. Then add salt, pepper and a couple of drops of olive oil to taste.

3. Bake for 15 minutes at 4000F in an air fryer (check every 5 minutes).

4. Serve with potatoes, herbal butter and a new salad.

5. Until it's creamy, whip the butter.

6. Add the same lemon juice and the herbs described previously.

### 87.Breaded Fish with Tartar Sauce
Preparation Time: 15 Minutes

Cooking Time: 20 Minutes

Servings: 2-4

### Ingredients:

- 1 lb of hake fillet
- 4 garlic cloves, crushed
- Juice of 2 lemons
- Salt and black pepper
- Beaten eggs
- Wheat flour
- Vegetable oil for frying

### Sauce:

- 3 oz. green olives
- 3 tbsp. chopped onion
- 1 garlic clove, crushed
- Parsley and chives
- 5 tbsp. soy sauce
- ½ can of cream
- 3 tbsp. of dijon mustard
- 1 tbsp. of tomato sauce
- 4 tbsp. mayonnaise

### Tartar sauce:

- ½ lb chopped pickles

## Directions:

1. Season the fillets with salt, pepper, garlic, and lemon juice, let them taste for at least 30 minutes.

2. Pass the wheat, egg and wheat again.

3. Fry them in the air fryer at 4000F for 25 minutes.

4. Mix all the ingredients in a bowl. 5. Serve with the fillets.

### 88. Milanese Fish Fillet

Preparation Time: 10 Minutes

Cooking Time: 30 Minutes

Servings: 2-3

### Ingredients:

- 1 lb of fish fillet of your choice
- Salt
- 2 garlic cloves, crushed
- 3 eggs Wheat flour
- Oil for frying

### Directions:

1. Wash and season the fish fillets with garlic and salt.

2. If you want, you can add the juice of a lemon.

3. Beat the egg whites until stiff and add the egg yolks.

4. Pass the fish fillets, one at a time, in the wheat flour and then pass them over the beaten eggs in the snow.

5. Fry in the air fryer at 4000F for 25 minutes or until they are golden brown.

### 89. Sole with White Wine

Preparation Time: 10 Minutes

Cooking Time: 35 Minutes

Servings: 4-6

### Ingredients:

- 3 lbs of sole fillets
- 5 ¼ oz. of butter
- 1 glass of white wine
- Wheat flour
- Salt black pepper thyme

## Directions:

1. Season the fillet with both the wheat flour and pass it on.

2. For 20 minutes or until brown, put in an air fryer at 4000F. In a preheated clay pan, reserve this fish.

3. In the butter, toast a tablespoon of flour.

4. Add the wine to taste, with salt, pepper and thyme. Let everything cook for another three minutes, stirring constantly. Pour the sole over and eat.

### 90.Golden Fish with Shrimps
Preparation Time: 10 Minutes

Cooking Time: 30 Minutes

Servings: 2-3

## Ingredients:

- 1 large golden fish
- 1 lb of shrimp onion
- tomato
- Pepper
- lemon
- olive oil
- Butter
- green smell parsley

## Directions:

1. Clean the complete golden and season with lemon, black pepper to taste and salt, the same with the prawns.

2. Leave for 1 hour after seasoning.

3. Place the fish on this plate, add the shrimp to the fish's belly, and tie it with a line. Line a plate with aluminum foil and grease with butter.

4. On top of the gold, put the onion rings, tomatoes and peppers and the green odor with the parsley and use it with plenty of oil.

5. Cover the tray with aluminum foil and bake for 35 minutes at 4000F in the air fryer.

6. With white rice, serve.

### 91.Stroganoff Cod
Preparation Time: 5 Minutes

Cooking Time: 35 Minutes

Servings: 4-6

### Ingredients:
- 1 lb of cod
- 3 tbsp. olive oil
- 2 garlic cloves, minced
- 2 ¼ lb of chopped onion
- 4 ½ lb of skinless tomatoes
- Salt to taste
- ½ cup of brandy
- Oregano, rosemary and black pepper to taste.
- 1 package of chopped green aroma
- 1 cup grated cheese
- 2 ¼ lb of fresh mushrooms cut into chips
- 1 can of sour cream
- 1 large golden fish
- 1 lb of shrimp onion tomato
- Pepper lemon olive oil
- Butter green smell parsley

### Directions:

1. Soak the cod in water the day before, boil and crumble all the meat. Reserve. Reserve.

2. In olive oil, saute the onion and garlic. Add the tomatoes that have been chopped and boil until separated. Remove. Remove!

3. Season with salt, oregano, rosemary and black pepper. Blend with the cod and apply the brandy. Add the mushrooms and the green odor.

4. Put it in an air-fryer for 10 minutes at 3200. Taking the fryer out of the air; add the grated cheese and sour cream.

5. Mix well with white rice and serve.

## 92.Cod Balls

Preparation Time: 10 Minutes

Cooking Time: 15 Minutes

Servings: 2-4

**Ingredients**:

- ½ lb salted and grated cod
- 3 cups boiled and squeezed potatoes
- 1 tbsp. of wheat flour
- Salt and black pepper to taste
- 3 eggs
- 2 tbsp. chopped green aroma

**Directions:**

1. In a bowl, mix all the ingredients well.

2. Form the balls with your hands.

3. Fry in the air fryer at 4000F for 30 minutes or until golden brown.

## 93.Lobster Bang Bang

Preparation Time: 15 Minutes

Cooking Time: 20 Minutes

Servings: 4

Ingredients:

- 1 cup cornstarch
- ¼ teaspoon Sriracha powder
- ¼ cup mayonnaise
- ¼ cup sweet chili sauce
- 4 lbs Lobsters

Directions:

1. In a big bowl, combine corn-starch and Sriracha powder.

2. Dredge lobsters with this mixture.

3. Place lobsters in the air fryer.

4. Choose an air fry setting.

5. Cook at 400 degrees F for 7 minutes per side.

6. Mix the mayo and chili sauce.

7. Serve shrimp with sauce.

## 94.Honey Glazed Salmon
Preparation Time: 10 Minutes

Cooking Time: 35 Minutes

Servings: 1

Ingredients:

- ¼ cup soy sauce
- ½ cup honey

- 1 tablespoon lemon juice
- 1 oz. orange juice
- 1 tablespoon brown sugar
- 1 teaspoon olive oil
- 1 tablespoon red wine vinegar
- 1 scallion, chopped
- 1 clove garlic, minced
- Salt and pepper to taste
- 1 salmon fillet

## Directions:

1. Mix all the ingredients except salt, pepper and salmon.

2. Place mixture in a pan over medium heat.

3. Bring to a boil.

4. Reduce heat.

5. Simmer for 15 minutes.

6. Turn off heat and transfer sauce to a bowl.

7. Sprinkle salt and pepper on both sides of the salmon.

8. Add salmon to the air fryer.

9. Select grill function.

## 95.Crispy Fish Fillet

Preparation Time: 10 Minutes

Cooking Time: 30 Minutes

Servings: 2

## Ingredients:

- 2 cod fillets
- 1 teaspoon Old Bay seasoning
- Salt and pepper to taste
- ½ cup all-purpose flour

- 1 egg, beaten
- 2 cups breadcrumbs

**Directions:**

1. Sprinkle both sides of cod with Old Bay seasoning, salt and pepper.

2. Coat with flour, dip in egg and dredge with breadcrumbs.

3. Add fish to the air fryer.

4. Select air fry setting.

5. Cook at 400 degrees F for 5 to 6 minutes per side.

## 96.Garlic Butter Lobster Tails

Preparation Time: 10 Minutes

Cooking Time: 15 Minutes

Servings: 2

**Ingredients:**

- 2 lobster tails
- 2 cloves garlic, minced
- 2 tablespoons butter
- 1 teaspoon lemon juice
- 1 teaspoon chopped chives
- Salt to taste

**Directions:**

1. Butterfly the lobster tails.

2. Place the meat on top of the shell.

3. Mix the remaining ingredients in a bowl.

4. Add lobster tails inside the air fryer.

5. Set it to air fry.

6. Spread garlic butter on the meat.

7. Cook at 380 degrees F for 5 minutes.

8. Spread more butter on top.

9. Cook for another 2 to 3 minutes.

## 97.Pesto Fish

Preparation Time: 10 Minutes

Cooking Time: 15 Minutes

Servings: 4

**Ingredients:**

- 1 tablespoon olive oil
- 4 fish fillets
- Salt and pepper to taste
- 1 cup olive oil
- 3 cloves garlic
- 1 ½ cups fresh basil leaves
- 2 tablespoons Parmesan cheese, grated
- 3 tablespoons pine nuts

**Directions:**

1. Drizzle olive oil over fish fillets and season with salt and pepper.

2. Add remaining ingredients to a food processor.

3. Pulse until smooth.

4. Transfer pesto to a bowl and set aside.

5. Add fish to the air fryer.

6. Select grill setting.

7. Cook at 320 degrees F for 5 minutes per side.

8. Spread pesto on top of the fish before serving.

## 98.Mozzarella Spinach Quiche

Prep time: 10 min

Cook time: 45 min

Yield: 6 servings

**Ingredients:**

- 4 eggs
- 10 oz. frozen spinach, thawed
- 1/2 cup mozzarella cheese, shredded
- 1/4 cup parmesan cheese, grated
- 8 oz. mushrooms, sliced
- 2 oz. feta cheese, crumbled
- 1 cup almond milk
- 1 garlic clove, minced
- Pepper
- Salt

## Directions:

44. Spray a pie dish with cooking spray and set it aside.
45. Insert wire rack in rack position 6. Select bake, set temperature 350 f, timer for 45 minutes. Press start to preheat the oven.
46. Spray medium pan with cooking spray and heat over medium heat.
47. Add garlic, mushrooms, pepper, and salt in a pan and sauté for 5 minutes.
48. Add spinach to the pie dish, then add sautéed mushroom on top of spinach.
49. Sprinkle feta cheese over spinach and mushroom.
50. In a bowl, whisk eggs, parmesan cheese, and almond milk.
51. Pour egg mixture over spinach and mushroom, then sprinkle shredded mozzarella cheese and bake for 45 minutes.
52. Sliced and serve.

## 99.Cheesy Zucchini Quiche

Total time: 1 hour 10 min

Prep time: 10 min

Cook time: 60 min

Yield: 8 servings

**Ingredients:**

- 2 eggs
- 2 cups cheddar cheese, shredded
- 1 1/2 cup almond milk
- Pepper
- Salt
- 2 lbs. zucchini, sliced

**Directions:**

1. Set aside and oil the quiche pan with cooking oil.
2. Wire rack insertion at rack position 6. Pick bake, set temperature to 375 f, 60-minute timer. To preheat the oven, press start.
3. With pepper and salt, season the zucchini and set aside for 30 minutes.
4. Mix the almond milk, spice, and salt with the eggs in a big cup.
5. Stir well and Mix sliced cheddar cheese.
6. Arrange slices of zucchini in a plate of quiche.
7. Pour the combination of eggs over the slices of zucchini and scatter with shredded cheese. For 60 minutes, roast.
8. Enjoy and serve.

## 100.Healthy Asparagus Quiche

Total time: 1 hour 10 min

Prep time: 10 min

Cook time: 60 min

Yield: 6 servings

**Ingredients:**

- 5 eggs, beaten
- 1 cup almond milk

- 15 asparagus spears, cut ends then cut asparagus in half
- 1 cup Swiss cheese, shredded
- 1/4 tsp. thyme
- 1/4 tsp. white pepper
- 1/4 tsp. salt

## Directions:

Grease quiche pan with cooking spray and set aside.

Insert wire rack in rack position 6. Select bake, set temperature 350 f, timer for 60 minutes. Press start to preheat the oven.

In a bowl, whisk together eggs, thyme, white pepper, almond milk, and salt.

Arrange asparagus in quiche pan, then pour egg mixture over asparagus. Sprinkle with shredded cheese.

Bake for 60 minutes.

Sliced and serve.

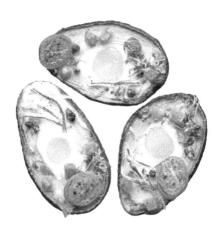

## Conclusion

Before you know how to use an Air Fryer, you need to make some plans before using it and take some steps accordingly. Such as getting an amazing recipe book to cook your food using an air fryer. This book will surely help you with that as it has covered a delicious range of air fryer recipes.

# The Air Fryer Recipes

How to Prepare Easy and Healthy Recipes for Quick And Easy Meals

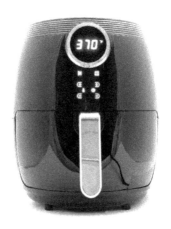

## Introduction

In the frying process, the Air Fryer is nothing but a groundbreaking invention and is a user-friendly device. It is essentially a frying machine that can use hot air to fry, bake or roast food and does not require any oil, although it also does not apply any oil to food. This ensures that the food that you fry stays free of calories and oil.

The Air Fryer lets you cook, roast, barbecue, and steam healthier, easier, and more effectively. As many others around the world do, we hope you enjoy using the Air Fryer, and the recipes inside inspire you to cook healthy, well-balanced meals for you and your family.

# Air Fryer Recipes

## 1.Mini Veggie Quiche Cups

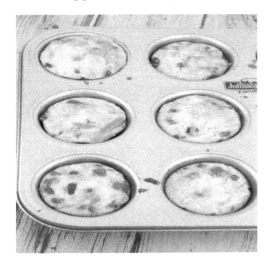

Total time: 30 min

Prep time: 10 min

Cook time: 20 min

Yield: 12 servings

### Ingredients:

- 8 eggs
- 3/4 cup cheddar cheese, shredded
- 10 oz. frozen spinach, chopped
- 1/4 cup onion, chopped
- 1/4 cup mushroom, diced
- 1/4 cup bell pepper, diced

### Directions:

53. Spray 12 cups muffin pan with cooking spray and set aside.
54. Insert wire rack in rack position 6. Select bake, set temperature 375 f, timer for 20 minutes. Press start to preheat the oven.
55. Add all ingredients into the mixing bowl and beat until combine.

56. Pour egg mixture into the prepared muffin pan and bake for 20 minutes.

57. Serve and enjoy.

## 2.Lemon Blueberry Muffins

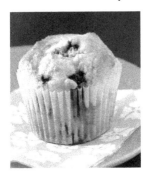

Total time: 35 min

Prep time: 10 min

Cook time: 25 min

Yield: 12 servings

**Ingredients:**

- 2 eggs
- 1 tsp. baking powder
- 5 drops stevia
- 1/4 cup butter, melted
- 1 cup heavy whipping cream
- 2 cups almond flour
- 1/4 tsp. lemon zest
- 1/2 tsp. lemon extract
- 1/2 cup fresh blueberries

**Directions:**

1. Spray the muffin pan with 12 cups of cooking spray and set it aside.

2. Wire rack insertion at rack position 6. Pick bake, set temperature to 350 f, 25-minute timer. To preheat the oven, press start.

3. Whisk the eggs together in a mixing dish.

4. Apply the remaining ingredients to the eggs and combine until well mixed.

5. In the prepared muffin tin, add flour and bake for 25 minutes.

6. Enjoy and serve.

7.

## 3.Baked Breakfast Donuts

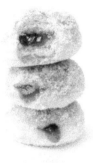

Total time: 30 min

Prep time: 10 min

Cook time: 20 min

Yield: 6 servings

**Ingredients:**

- 4 eggs
- 1/3 cup almond milk
- 1 tbsp. liquid stevia
- 3 tbsp. cocoa powder
- 1/4 cup coconut oil
- 1/3 cup coconut flour
- 1/2 tsp. baking soda
- 1/2 tsp. baking powder
- 1/2 tsp. instant coffee

**Directions:**

1. Spray donut pan with cooking spray and set aside.

2. Insert wire rack in rack position 6. Select bake, set temperature 350 f, timer for 20 minutes. Press start to preheat the oven.

3. Add all ingredients into the mixing bowl and mix until well combined.

4. Pour batter into the donut pan and bake for 20 minutes.

5. Serve and enjoy.

### 4. Blueberry Almond Muffins

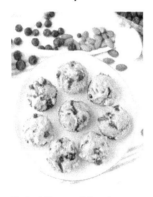

Total time: 25 min

Prep time: 10 min

Cook time: 15 min

Yield: 8 servings

**Ingredients:**

- 1 egg
- 5 drops liquid stevia
- 1/4 tsp. vanilla extract
- 3/4 cup heavy cream
- 1/4 cup butter
- 1/2 cup fresh blueberries
- 1/2 tsp. baking soda
- 1/4 tsp. baking powder

- 2 1/2 cup almond flour
- 1/2 tsp. salt

**Directions:**

59. Spray 8 cups muffin pan with cooking spray and set aside.

60. Insert wire rack in rack position 6. Select bake, set temperature 375 f, timer for 15 minutes. Press start to preheat the oven.

61. In a bowl, mix together almond flour, salt, and baking powder.

62. In a large bowl, whisk together egg, butter, vanilla, stevia, baking soda, and heavy cream.

63. Add almond flour mixture into the egg mixture and stir to combine.

64. Pour batter into the muffin pan and bake for 15 minutes.

65. Serve and enjoy.

**5.Feta Broccoli Frittata**

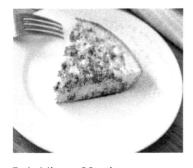

Total time: 30 min

Prep time: 10 min

Cook time: 20 min

Yield: 4 servings

**Ingredients:**

- 10 eggs
- 2 oz. feta cheese, crumbled
- 2 cups broccoli florets, chopped

- 1 tomato, diced
- 1 tsp. black pepper
- 1 tsp. salt

**Directions:**

1. Grease baking dish with butter and set aside.

2. Insert wire rack in rack position 6. Select bake, set temperature 390 f, timer for 20 minutes. Press start to preheat the oven.

3. In a bowl, whisk eggs, pepper, and salt. Add veggies and stir well.

4. Pour egg mixture into the baking dish and sprinkle with crumbled cheese.

5. Bake for 20 minutes.

6. Serve and enjoy.

### 6.Creamy Spinach Quiche

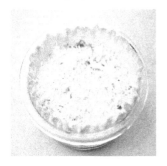

Total time: 45 min

Prep time: 10 min

Cook time: 35 min

Yield: 6 servings

**Ingredients:**

- 10 eggs
- 1 cup heavy cream
- 1 tbsp. butter
- 1/4 cup fresh scallions, minced
- 1 cup cheddar cheese, shredded
- 1/4 tsp. pepper
- 1/4 tsp. salt
- 1 cup fresh spinach
- 1 cup of coconut milk

**Directions:**

1. Spray 9*13-inch baking pan with cooking spray and set aside.
2. Insert wire rack in rack position 6. Select bake, set temperature 350 f, timer for 35 minutes. Press start to preheat the oven.
3. In a bowl, whisk eggs, cream, coconut milk, pepper, and salt.

4. Pour egg mixture into the baking pan and sprinkle with spinach, scallions, and cheese.

5. Bake for 35 minutes.

6. Serve and enjoy.

## 7.Turkey and Quinoa Stuffed Peppers

Total time: 50 min

Prep time: 15 min

Cook time: 35 min

Yield: 6 servings

**Ingredients:**

- 3 large red bell peppers
- 2 tsp. Chopped fresh rosemary
- 2 tbsp. Chopped fresh parsley
- 3 tbsp. Chopped pecans, toasted
- 2 tbsp. Extra virgin olive oil
- ½ cup chicken stock
- ½ lb. Fully cooked smoked turkey sausage, diced
- ½ tsp. Salt
- 2 cups water
- 1 cup uncooked quinoa

**Directions:**

1. Place a large saucepan on a high flame and add salt, water and quinoa. Just get it to a boil.

2. Reduce the fire to a simmer after boiling, cover and cook until all the water is consumed for about 15 minutes.

3. Switch off the fire and let it stand for another 5 minutes. Uncover the quinoa.

4. Lengthwise, break the peppers in half and remove the membranes and seeds. Add the peppers to another boiling pot of water, cook for 5 minutes, rinse and discard the water.

5. Grease a 13 x 9 baking dish and preheat the oven to 350.

6. Put the boiling bell pepper on the prepared baking dish, fill the quinoa mixture evenly and pop it into the oven.

7. For 15 minutes, roast.

## 8.Curried Chicken, Chickpeas and Raito Salad

Prep time: 10 minutes

Cook time: 30 minutes

Yield: 5 servings

**Ingredients:**

- 1 cup red grapes, halved
- 3-4 cups rotisserie chicken, meat coarsely shredded
- 2 tbsp. Cilantro
- 1 cup plain yogurt
- 2 medium tomatoes, chopped
- 1 tsp. ground cumin
- 1 tbsp. Curry powder
- 2 tbsp. Vegetable oil
- 1 tbsp. Minced peeled ginger
- 1 tbsp. Minced garlic
- 1 medium onion, chopped
- Chickpeas ingredients:
- ¼ tsp. Cayenne
- ½ tsp. Turmeric
- 1 tsp. ground cumin
- 1 19-oz can chickpeas, rinsed, drained and patted dry

- 1 tbsp. Vegetable oil
- Topping and ratio ingredients:
- ½ cup sliced and toasted almonds
- 2 tbsp. Chopped mint
- 2 cups cucumber, peeled, cored and chopped
- 1 cup plain yogurt

## Directions:

1. To make the chicken salad, on medium-low fire, place a medium nonstick saucepan and heat oil.

2. Sauté ginger, garlic and onion for 5 minutes or until softened while stirring occasionally.

3. Add 1 ½ tsp. Salt, cumin and curry. Sauté for two minutes.

4. Increase fire to medium-high and add tomatoes. Stirring frequently, cook for 5 minutes.

5. Pour sauce into a bowl, mix in chicken, cilantro and yogurt. Stir to combine and let it stand to cool to room temperature.

6. To make the chickpeas, on a nonstick fry pan, heat oil for 3 minutes.

7. Add chickpeas and cook for a minute while stirring almost continually.

8. Add ¼ tsp. Salt, cayenne, turmeric and cumin. Stir to mix well and cook for two minutes or until sauce is dried.

9. Transfer to a bowl and let it cool to room temperature.

10. To make the ratio, mix ½ tsp. salt, mint, cucumber and yogurt. Stir thoroughly to combine and dissolve the salt.

11. To assemble, in four 16-oz lidded jars or bowls, layer the following: curried chicken, ratio, chickpeas, and garnish with almonds.

12. You can make this recipe one day ahead and refrigerate for 6 hours before serving.

# 9.Balsamic Vinaigrette on Roasted Chicken

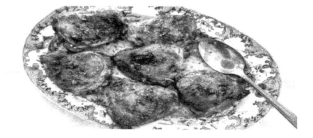

Total time: 1 hour 10 min

Prep time: 10 min

Cook time: 60 min

Yield: 8 servings

**Ingredients:**

- 1 tbsp. Chopped fresh parsley
- 1 tsp. Lemon zest
- ½ cup low-salt chicken broth
- One 4-lb whole chicken, cut into pieces
- Freshly ground black pepper
- Salt
- 2 tbsp. Olive oil
- 2 garlic cloves, chopped
- 2 tbsp. Fresh lemon juice
- 2 tbsp. Dijon mustard
- ¼ cup balsamic vinegar

**Directions:**

1. Whisk together the pepper, salt, olive oil, garlic, lemon juice, mustard and vinegar in a small cup.

2. Combine the above mixture and the chicken parts in a re-sealable bag. Refrigerate for at least 2 hours or a whole day and

marinate. Make sure that the bag is turned upside-down sometimes.

3. Grease a baking dish and preheat the 400 ° f oven.

4. Place marinated pieces of chicken on a baking dish and popped them into the oven.

5. Roast the chicken for an hour or until fully baked. Cover with foil if the chicken is browned and not yet completely baked, and finish cooking.

6. Take the chicken out of the oven and pass it to a serving dish.

7. Garnish with parsley and, before eating, drizzle with lemon juice.

## 10.Chicken Pasta Parmesan

Total time: 30 min

Prep time: 10 min

Cook time: 20 min

Yield: 1servings

**Ingredients:**

- ½ cup cooked whole-wheat spaghetti
- 1 oz. Reduced-fat mozzarella cheese, grated
- ¼ cup prepared marinara sauce
- 2 tbsp. Seasoned dry breadcrumbs
- 4 oz. Skinless chicken breast
- 1 tbsp. Olive oil

**Directions:**

1. On medium-high fire, place an ovenproof skillet and heat oil.

2. Pan Fry chicken for 3 to 5 minutes per side or until cooked through.

3. Pour marinara sauce, stir and continue cooking for 3 minutes.

4. Turn off fire, add mozzarella and breadcrumbs on top.

5. Pop into a preheated broiler on high and broil for 10 minutes or until breadcrumbs are browned, and mozzarella is melted.

6. Remove from broiler, serve and enjoy.

## 11. Chicken and White Bean

Total time: 1 hour 20 min

Prep time: 10 min

Cook time: 70 min

Yield: 6 servings

**Ingredients:**

- 2 tbsp. Fresh cilantro, chopped
- 2 cups grated low-fat Monterey jack cheese
- 3 cups water
- 1/8 tsp. Cayenne pepper
- 2 tsp. Pure Chile powder
- 2 tsp. ground cumin
- 1 4-oz can chop green chills
- 1 cup corn kernels
- 2 15-oz cans white beans, drained and rinsed
- 2 garlic cloves
- 1 medium onion, diced
- 2 tbsp. Extra virgin olive oil
- 1 lb. Chicken breasts, boneless and skinless

**Directions:**

1. Slice the chicken breasts into 1/2-inch chunks and season with salt and pepper.

2. Place a large anti-adhesive fry pan and heat oil on high fire.

3. Sauté the pieces of chicken for 3 to 4 minutes, or until finely browned.

4. Reduce the heat to mild and add the onion and garlic.

5. Cook for 5 to 6 minutes or until it is translucent with onions.

6. Stir in the sugar, peppers, chilies, maize, and beans. Just get it to a boil.

7. When baked, boil slowly and proceed to simmer for an hour, uncovered.

8. Garnish it with a dash of cilantro and a tablespoon of cheese to serve.

## 36. Chicken Pad Thai

Total time: 20 min

Prep time: 10 min

Cook time: 10 min

Yield: 6 servings

**Ingredients:**

- 2 medium sized carrots, julienned
- 1 12oz package broccoli slaw
- 5 green onions, chopped
- 5 tbsp. Fresh cilantro, chopped
- ½ tbsp. Coconut vinegar
- 4 tbsp. Fresh lime juice
- 1 tbsp. Coconut amines
- 3 tbsp. Fish sauce
- 5 cloves garlic, crushed
- 2 tbsp. Extra virgin coconut oil
- 1 ½ lb. Organic chicken meat, cut into chunks

**Directions:**

1. Over medium pressure, heat the skillet and apply the coconut oil.

2. For one minute, sauté the garlic and onion.

3. Add the chicken, then simmer for 5 minutes.

4. Placed the amines in the coconut, fish sauce, vinegar, and lime juice. Increase the heat and boil until the chicken is cooked thoroughly.

5. Add the carrots and broccoli slaw. Constantly stir until the vegetables become tender.

6. Garnish with green onions and cilantro.

## 12. Chicken Thighs with Butternut Squash

Total time: 40 min

Prep time: 10 min

Cook time: 30 min

Yield: 6 servings

**Ingredients:**

- 3 cups butternut squash, cubed
- 6 boneless chicken thighs
- A sprig of fresh sage, chopped
- 1 tbsp. Olive oil
- Salt and pepper to taste

**Directions:**

1. Preheat the 425°f oven.

2. Sauté the butternut squash in a skillet and season with salt and pepper to taste. Remove from the skillet after the squash is cooked and put aside.

3. Using the same pan, add oil and cook the chicken thighs on either side for 10 minutes.

4. Season with salt and pepper and return the squash to the mixture.

5. Take the skillet from the stove and cook it for 15 minutes in the oven.

6. Serving and enjoying!

## 13.Cajun Rice & Chicken

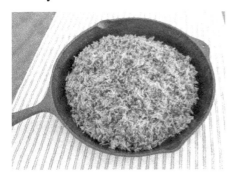

Total time: 30 min

Prep time: 10 min

Cook time: 20 min

Yield: 6 servings

**Ingredients:**

- 1 tablespoon oil
- 1 onion, diced
- 3 cloves of garlic, minced
- 1-pound chicken breasts, sliced
- 1 tablespoon Cajun seasoning
- 1 tablespoon tomato paste
- 3 cups chicken broth
- 1 ½ cups brown rice, rinsed
- 1 bell pepper, chopped

**Directions:**

1. Place a heavy-bottomed pot on medium-high fire and heat for 2 minutes.
2. Add oil and heat for a minute.
3. Sauté the onion and garlic until fragrant.

4. Stir in the chicken breasts and season with Cajun seasoning.

5. Continue cooking for 3 minutes.

6. Add the tomato paste, rice, and chicken broth. Bring to a boil while stirring to dissolve the tomato paste.

7. Once boiling, lower fire to a simmer, cover and cook until liquid is fully absorbed around 15 minutes.

8. Turn off the fire and let it stand for another 5 minutes before serving.

## 14. Vegetable Lover's Chicken Soup

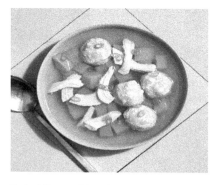

Total time: 30 min

Prep time: 10 min

Cook time: 20 min

Yield: 4 servings

**Ingredients:**

- 1 ½ cups baby spinach
- 2 tbsp. Orzo (tiny pasta)
- ¼ cup dry white wine
- 1 14oz low sodium chicken broth
- 2 plum tomatoes, chopped
- 1/8 tsp. Salt

- ½ tsp. Italian seasoning
- 1 large shallot, chopped
- 1 small zucchini, diced
- 8-oz chicken tenders
- 1 tbsp. Extra virgin olive oil

**Directions:**

1. In a large saucepan, heat oil over medium heat and add the chicken. Stir occasionally for 8 minutes until browned. Transfer in a plate. Set aside.

2. In the same saucepan, add the zucchini, Italian seasoning, shallot and salt and often stir until the vegetables are softened around 4 minutes.

3. Add the tomatoes, wine, broth and orzo and increase the heat to high to bring the mixture to boil. Reduce the heat and simmer.

4. Add the cooked chicken and stir in the spinach last.

5. Serve hot.

6.

## 15.Coconut Flour Cheesy Garlic Biscuits

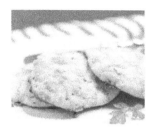

Total time: 20 min

Prep time: 10 min

Cook time: 10 min

Yield: 4 servings

### Ingredients:

- 1/3 cup of coconut flour
- 1/2 teaspoon of baking powder
- 1/2 teaspoon of garlic powder
- 1 large egg
- 1/4 cup of unsalted butter, melted and divided
- 1/2 cup of shredded sharp Cheddar cheese
- 1 scallion, sliced

### Directions:

1. In a broad dish, combine the coconut flour, baking powder, and garlic powder together.

2. Add the egg, half of the melted butter, the scallions and the cheddar cheese. In a 6 'circular baking tray, pour the mixture. Place it within the Air Fryer frame.

3. Set the temperature to 320 degrees F and change the 12-minute timer.

4. Remove and allow to cool fully from the pan to eat. Slice into four pieces and pour on any remaining butter.

## 16. Radish Chips

Total time: 20 min

Prep time: 10 min

Cook time: 10 min

Yield: 4 servings

**Ingredients:**

- 2 cups of water
- 1-pound of radishes
- 1/4 teaspoon of onion powder
- 1/4 teaspoon of paprika
- 1/2 teaspoon of garlic powder
- 2 tablespoons of coconut oil, melted

**Directions:**

1. Place water on a stovetop and bring to a boil in a medium saucepan.

2. Cut the top and bottom of each radish, then thinly and finely slice each radish with a mandolin. You could use the slicing blade in the food processor for this point, too.

3. Place the radish slices for 5 minutes in boiling water, or until they are translucent. To retain additional moisture, remove it from the bath and place it in a clean kitchen towel.

4. Place the radish chips with the remaining ingredients in a large bowl and season until completely coated with grease. Place the radish chips inside the Air Fryer basket.

5. Set the timer for 5 minutes and turn to 320° F.

6. Two or three times, shake a basket during the cooking process.

## 17. Flatbread

Total time: 20 min

Prep time: 10 min

Cook time: 10 min

Yield:  4 servings

**Ingredients:**

- 1 cup of shredded mozzarella cheese
- 1/4 cup of blanched finely ground almond flour
- 1 ounce of full-Fat: cream cheese, softened

**Directions:**

1. In a large, microwave-safe bowl, melt the mozzarella for 30 seconds. Stir in the almond flour until it is smooth, then apply the cream cheese. Continue to mix until the dough emerges, softly kneading it if necessary with wet hands.

2. "Break the dough into two parts and stretch to 1/4" thickness between two parchments. To fit the Air Fryer tray, cut another slice of parchment.

3. On your parchment and in the Air Fryer, place a slice of flatbread and work in two batches if appropriate.

4. Set the temperature to 320 degrees F and set a seven-minute timer.

5. Turn halfway through the cooking time on the flat-bread. Serve hot.

**18. Avocado Fries**

Total time: 20 min

Prep time: 10 min

Cook time: 10 min

Yield:  4 servings

**Ingredients:**

- 2 medium avocados
- 1-ounce of pork rinds, finely ground

**Directions:**

1. Cut out half the avocado from each one. Smash the fuselage. Gently cut the peel, then break the beef into 1/4-inch-thick slices.

2. In a medium cup, place the pork rinds and press each slice of avocado onto the pork rinds to cover them entirely.

3. Set the temperature to 350° F and set five minutes for the timer.

4. Serve it hot.

## 19. Pita-Style Chips

Total time: 20 min

Prep time: 10 min

Cook time: 10 min

Yield:  4 servings

**Ingredients:**

- 1 cup of shredded mozzarella cheese
- ½ ounce of pork rinds, finely ground
- ¼ cup of blanched finely ground almond flour
- 1 large egg

**Directions:**

1. In a large microwave and microwave dish, place the mozzarella for 30 seconds or until it has melted. Attach the remaining ingredients and stir to a smooth finish; the dough forms into a ball easily. If the dough is too hard, microwave it for 15 seconds.

2. Roll out the dough between two sheets of parchment into a large rectangle and then use a knife to cut triangle-shaped chips. Put the Air Fryer chips in the basket.

3. Set the temperature to 350° F and set five minutes for the timer.

4. The chips will be golden in color and sturdy when done. When they cool down, they'll be even firmer.

## 20. Roasted Eggplant

Total time: 20 min

Prep time: 10 min

Cook time: 10 min

Yield: 4 servings

**Ingredients:**

- 1 large eggplant
- 2 tablespoons of olive oil
- 1/4 teaspoon of salt
- 1/2 teaspoon of garlic powder

**Directions:**

1. Split the top and bottom of the eggplant. Break the eggplant into thick, thin strips.
2. Using olive oil to brush the slices and dust with salt and garlic powder. Place the bits in the jar with the eggplant.
3. Set the temperature to 390° F for 15 minutes and change the timer.
4. Serve promptly and enjoy yourself!

**21.Parmesan-Herb Focaccia Bread**

Total time: 20 min

Prep time: 10 min

Cook time: 10 min

Yield: 4 servings

**Ingredients:**

- 1 cup of shredded mozzarella cheese
- 1 ounce of full-Fat: cream cheese
- 1 cup of blanched finely ground almond flour
- 1/4 cup of ground golden flaxseed
- 1/4 cup of grated Parmesan cheese

- 1/2 teaspoon of baking soda
- 2large eggs
- 1/2 teaspoon of garlic powder
- 1/4 teaspoon of dried basil
- 1/4 teaspoon of dried rosemary
- 2 tablespoons of salted butter, melted and divided

**Directions:**

1. Place the mozzarella, cream cheese, and almond flour for 1 minute in a large microwave-safe bowl and microwave. Parmesan, flaxseed, and baking soda are added, and stir until the ball is smooth. If the mixture cools so fast, so it would be impossible to combine. When needed, return to the microwave to rewarm for 10-15 seconds.

2. The substitute ducks. To Mix them to the full, you can need to use your hands. Only keep frying, and then add them to the batter.

3. Mix the basil and rosemary with the powdered garlic dough and knead them into the dough. In a round baking pan, grease 1 tablespoon of melted butter. Similarly, put the dough in the pan. Place the pan in an Air Fryer basket.

4. Set the temperature to 400 degrees F and for 10 minutes, change the timer.

5. If the bread begins to get too black, cover with foil after 7 minutes.

6. Remove and cool for at least 30 minutes, then combine and eat with the remaining butter.

**22. Quick and Easy Home Fries**

Total time: 20 min

Prep time: 10 min

Cook time: 10 min

Yield: 4 servings

**Ingredients:**

- 1 medium jicama, peeled
- 1 tablespoon of coconut oil, melted
- 1/4 teaspoon of ground black pepper
- ½ teaspoon of pink Himalayan salt
- 1 medium green bell pepper, seeded and diced
- 1/2 medium white onion, peeled and diced

**Directions:**

1. Split the cubed jicama. Put it in a large bowl and mix until seasoned with coconut oil. Sprinkle with salt and pepper. Place the pepper and onion in a jar with the fryer.

2. Adjust the temperature and set a 10-minute timer to 400°F. Shake it three times before cooking it. Around the sides, Jicama will be smooth and dark and serve immediately.

**23. Jicama Fries**

Total time: 20 min

Prep time: 10 min

Cook time: 10 min

Yield: 4 servings

**Ingredients:**

- 1 small jicama, peeled
- 3/4 teaspoon of chili powder
- 1/4 teaspoon of garlic powder
- 1/4 teaspoon of onion powder
- 1/4 teaspoon of ground black pepper

**Directions:**

1. Break the jicama into cubes of 1'. Place in a large bowl and mix until coated with the coconut oil. Sprinkle with salt and pepper. In the fryer pan, put the pepper and onion.

2. Adjust the temperature and set a 10-minute timer to 400° F.

3. Shake two or three times before cooking. Jicama around the edges will be smooth and dark and will serve instantly.

## 24. Fried Green Tomatoes

Total time: 20 min

Prep time: 10 min

Cook time: 10 min

Yield: 4 servings

### Ingredients:

- 2 medium green tomatoes
- 1 large egg
- 1/4 cup of blanched finely ground almond flour
- 1/3 cup of grated Parmesan cheese

### Directions:

1. Break the tomatoes into 1/2-inch-thick slices. In a medium bowl, whisk the egg. In a large bowl, combine the almond flour and parmesan.

2. Dip each tomato slice into the egg, then dredge in the almond flour mixture and drop the slices in the basket of the Air Fryer.

3. Set the temperature to 400 degrees F and set a seven-minute timer.

4. Halfway through the duration of cooking, turn the slices. Serve immediately.

## 25. Fried Pickles

Total time: 20 min

Prep time: 10 min

Cook time: 10 min

Yield: 4 servings

### Ingredients:

- 1 tablespoon of coconut flour
- 1/3 cup of blanched finely ground almond flour
- 1teaspoon of chili powder
- 1/4 teaspoon of garlic powder
- 1 large egg
- 1 cup of sliced pickles

**Directions:**

1. In a medium dish, mix the coconut flour, almond meal, chili powder, and garlic powder.

2. Whisk the egg in a tiny mug.

3. Pat with a paper towel on each pickle and dunk in the egg. Then dredge in the mixture with flour. Put the pickles in the bowl for Air Fryer.

4. Switch to 400° F and set the timer for 5 minutes.

5. Flip the pickles halfway through the duration of preparation.

**26.Pork and Potatoes**

Preparation time: 5 minutes

Cooking time: 25 minutes

Servings: 4

**Ingredients:**

- 2 cups creamer potatoes, rinsed and dried
- 1 (1-pound) pork tenderloin, slice into 1-inch cubes
- 1 onion, red bell pepper, 2 garlic clover
- ½ teaspoon dried oregano
- 2 tablespoons low-sodium chicken broth

**Directions:**

1. To coat, toss the potatoes and olive oil.

2. Move the potatoes to the basket of an air fryer. For 15 minutes, bake.

3.  Combine the bacon, cabbage, tomato, red bell pepper, garlic, and oregano together.

4.  Drizzle the chicken broth with it. Place the bowl in the basket of an air fryer. During frying, roast and shake the basket once before the pork hits a meat thermometer of at least 145 ° f, and the potatoes are tender. Immediately serve.

## 27.Pork and Fruit Kebabs

Preparation time: 15 minutes

Cooking time: 9 to 12 minutes

Servings: 4

**Ingredients:**

- 1/3 cup apricot jam
- 2 tablespoons freshly squeezed lemon juice
- ½ teaspoon dried tarragon
- 1 (1-pound) pork tenderloin, slice into 1-inch cubes
- 4 plums, small apricots, pitted and halved

**Directions:**

1.  Combine the jam, lemon juice, tarragon and olive oil.

2.  To coat, add the pork and stir. Place it aside at room temperature for 10 minutes.

3.  Thread the bacon, plums, and apricots onto 4 metal skewers that fit into the air fryer, alternating the items. Rub with a combination of any leftover jelly. Discard every marinade that exists.

4.  In an air fryer, grill the kebabs for 9 to 12 minutes. Immediately serve.

## 28.Steak and Vegetable Kebabs

Preparation time: 15 minutes

Cooking time: 7 minutes

Servings: 4

**Ingredients:**

- 2 tablespoons balsamic vinegar
- ½ teaspoon dried marjoram
- ¾ pound round steak, cut into 1-inch pieces
- 1 cup red bell pepper, cherry tomatoes
- 16 button mushrooms

**Directions:**

1. Stir together the balsamic vinegar, olive oil, black pepper and marjoram.
2. To coat, add the steak and stir. Leave it to rest at room temperature for 9 minutes.
3. Thread the meat, red bell pepper, mushrooms and tomatoes onto 8 bamboo or metal skewers that match in the air fryer, rotating products.
4. Grill for 6 minutes in the air-fryer. Immediately serve.

**29.Spicy Grilled Steak**

Preparation time: 7 minutes

Cooking time: 9 minutes

Servings: 4

**Ingredients:**

- 2 tablespoons low-sodium salsa
- 1 tablespoon chipotle pepper, apple cider vinegar
- 1 teaspoon ground cumin
- 1/8 tsp. Red pepper flakes
- ¾ lb. Sirloin tip steak mildly pounded to about 1/3 inch thick

**Directions:**

1. Add chili, chipotle pepper, cider vinegar, cumin, black pepper and red pepper flakes. Scrub this mixture onto each steak piece on both sides. Let it stand at room temperature for 15 minutes.

2. In an air fryer, grill the steaks, two at a time, for 6 to 9 minutes.

3. To stay warm, put the steaks on a clean plate and cover them with aluminum foil. Repeat for the steaks that remain.

4. Thinly chop the steaks against the grain and serve.

### 30.Greek Vegetable Skillet
Preparation time: 10 minutes

Cooking time: 19 minutes

Servings: 4

### Ingredients:

- ½ pound 96 percent lean ground beef
- 2 medium tomatoes, garlic clove
- 2 cups fresh baby spinach
- 1/3 cup low-sodium beef broth
- 2 tablespoons crumbled low-sodium feta cheese, lemon juice

### Directions:

1. Crumble the beef in a 6-by-2-inch metal pan. Cook for 3 to 7 minutes in an air fryer, stirring once during frying until browned. Drain some fat or liquid out.

2. To the pan, add the tomatoes, 1 onion, and garlic. Air-fry for an additional 4 to 8 minutes.

3. Spinach, lemon juice, and beef broth are added. Air-fry for an additional 2 or 4 minutes.

4. Place the feta cheese on top of it and serve right away.

### 31.Light Herbed Meatballs
Preparation time: 10 minutes

Cooking time: 17 minutes

Servings: 24

### Ingredients:

- 2 garlic cloves, minced

- 1 slice low-sodium whole-wheat bread, crumbled

- 3 tablespoons 1 percent milk

- 1 teaspoon dried marjoram, basil

- 1-pound 96 percent lean ground beef

**Directions:**

1. Combine the onion, garlic, and olive oil in a 6-by-2-inch pan. For 2 to 4 minutes, air-fry.

2. Put the vegetables in a medium bowl and combine with the bread crumbs, milk, basil, and marjoram. Mix thoroughly.

3. Add some ground beef. Run the mixture softly but thoroughly with your hands until mixed. Shape about 24 (1-inch) meatballs into a meat mixture.

4. Bake the meatballs, in lots, for 12 to 17 minutes in the air-fryer basket. Immediately serve.

### 32. Brown Rice and Beef-Stuffed Bell Peppers

Preparation time: 10 minutes

Cooking time: 16 minutes

Servings: 4

**Ingredients:**

- ½ cup grated carrot

- 1 cup cooked brown rice

- 1 cup chopped cooked low-sodium roast beef

- 4 bell peppers, 2 medium beefsteak tomatoes, onion

- 1 teaspoon dried marjoram

**Directions**:

1. Strip the bell pepper tops from the stems and chop the tops.

2. Combine the chopped bell pepper, onion, carrot, and olive oil in a 6-by-2-inch pan. Cook for 4 minutes, or until the vegetables are soft and crispy.

3. To a medium bowl, shift the vegetable. Add the onions, brown rice, marjoram, and roast beef. Stir to blend.

4. Stuff the combination of the vegetables into the bell peppers. Place the bell peppers in the basket of an air fryer. Bake or until the peppers are tender and the filling is sweet, for 14 minutes.

5. Instantly serve.

### 33. Beef and Broccoli
Preparation time: 10 minutes

Cooking time: 18 minutes

Servings: 4

### Ingredients:

- ½ cup low-sodium beef broth

- 1 teaspoon low-sodium soy sauce

- 12 ounces sirloin strip steak, cut into 1-inch cubes

- 1 cup sliced cremini mushrooms, onion, ginger

- 2½ cups broccoli florets

### Directions:

1. Stir 2 tablespoons of cornstarch, beef broth, and soy sauce together.

2. Attach the beef and cover with a toss. Set aside at room temperature for 5 minutes.

3. Move the beef from the broth combination into a small metal bowl with a slotted spoon.

4. Attach the beef to the broccoli, cabbage, mushrooms, and ginger. Place the bowl in the air fryer and cook for 12 to 15 minutes or on a meat thermometer until the beef hits at least 145 ° f and the vegetables are tender.

5. Attach the reserved broth and simmer for another 2 to 3 minutes or until the sauce is ready to boil.

6. If needed, serve immediately over hot cooked brown rice.

### 34. Beef and Fruit Stir-Fry

Preparation time: 15 minutes

Cooking time: 11 minutes

Servings: 4

**Ingredients:**

- 12 ounces sirloin tip steak, thinly sliced
- 1 tablespoon lime juice, cornstarch
- 1 cup canned mandarin orange segments, pineapple chunks
- 1 teaspoon low-sodium soy sauce
- 2 scallions, white and green parts, sliced

**Directions:**

1. Mix the lime juice with the steak. Just put aside.

2. Combine 3 tablespoons of reserved orange mandarin juice, 3 tablespoons of reserved pineapple juice, soy sauce, and cornstarch thoroughly.

3. Dry the beef and place it in a medium-sized metal cup, reserving the juice. Stir the reserved juice into the mixture of the mandarin-pineapple juice. And put aside.

4. Add to the steak the olive oil and the scallions. Put the metal bowl in the air fryer and reheat for 3 to 4 minutes, or shake the basket once during the cooking, until the steak is almost cooked.

5. Stir in a blend of mandarin oranges, pineapple and milk. Cook for 3 to 7 more minutes, or until the sauce is bubbling and the beef on a meat thermometer is soft and reaches at least 145 ° f.

6. If needed, stir and serve over warm fried brown rice.

### 35.Perfect Garlic Butter Steak

Preparation time: 20 minutes

Cooking time: 12 minutes

Servings: 4

**Ingredients:**

- 2 rib-eye steaks

- Garlic butter:
- ½ cup softened butter
- 2 tbsp. Chopped fresh parsley
- 2 garlic cloves, minced
- 1 tsp. Worcestershire sauce

**Directions:**

1. Add each of the ingredients together to prepare the garlic butter.

2. Place the document on parchment. Roll it up and put it in the refrigerator.

3. Just let steaks remain at room temperature for 20 minutes.

4. Brush some of the grease, salt, and pepper with it.

5. Pre-heat up to 400 ° f (200 ° c) with your hot air fryer.

6. 12 minutes to cook, rotating halfway through the cooking process. Just serve.

7. Top the steaks with the garlic butter and let hang for 5 minutes.

8. Enjoy and Serve!

### 36.Crispy Pork Medallions
Preparation time: 20 minutes

Cooking time: 5 minutes

Servings: 2

**Ingredients:**

- 1 pork loin, 330 g, cut into 6 or 7 slices of 4 cm
- Asian marinade:
- 1 tsp. Salt reduced tamari sauce, olive oil
- 1 clementine juice
- 1 pinch cayenne pepper
- 2 cloves garlic, pressed

**Directions:**

1. Get the marinade prepared first. Combine all the ingredients in a dish. Salt the medallions gently, apply pepper and sprinkle with 1 tsp. About paprika. Place these in the marinade and turn them to soak them full many times. Cover with plastic wrap and marinate at room temperature for 1 hour.

2. Merge 1/3 of a cup of breadcrumbs, 1/2 of orange zest and 2 grams of parmesan cheese in a deep dish to prepare the covering.

3. Remove the marinade medallions and dry them on absorbent paper after the time for maceration has expired. Fill with mustard, and move on to the sheet that is crunchy. Lightly brush with oil.

4. Heat the air-fryer to 350 degrees F. Place the medallions in the basket with the fryer. Cook for five minutes, stir, and then bring it back in the fryer for another minute. Immediately serve.

### 37. Parmesan Meatballs

Preparation time: 10 minutes

Cooking time: 20 minutes

Servings: 6

**Ingredients:**

- 2 lbs. Ground beef
- 2 eggs
- 1 cup ricotta cheese
- 1/4 cup parmesan cheese shredded
- 1/2 cup panko breadcrumbs
- 1/4 cup basil chopped
- 1/4 cup parsley chopped
- 1 tablespoon fresh oregano chopped
- 2 teaspoon kosher salt
- 1 teaspoon ground fennel
- 1/2 teaspoon red pepper flakes
- 32 oz. spaghetti sauce, to serve

**Directions:**

1. In a bowl, carefully mix the beef with all the other meatball ingredients.

2. Create tiny meatballs out of this combination, then put them in the basket of the air fryer.

3. Click the Air Fry Oven control button and switch the knob to pick the bake mode.

4. To set the cooking time to 20 minutes, click the time button and change the dial once again.

5. Now press the temp button to set the temperature at 400 degrees f and rotate the dial.

6. When preheated, put the basket of meatballs in the oven and close the lid.

7. When baked, turn the meatballs halfway through and then start cooking.

8. On top, pour the spaghetti sauce.

9. Serve it hot.

## 38.Tricolor Beef Skewers

Preparation time: 10 minutes

Cooking time: 25 minutes

Servings: 4

**Ingredients:**

- 3 garlic cloves, minced
- 4 tablespoon rapeseed oil
- 1 cup cottage cheese, cubed
- 16 cherry tomatoes
- 2 tablespoon cider vinegar
- Large bunch thyme
- 1 ¼ lb. Boneless beef, diced

**Directions:**

1. Toss beef with all its thyme, oil, vinegar, and garlic.

2. Marinate the thyme beef for 2 hours in a closed container in the refrigerator.

3. Thread the marinated beef, cheese, and tomatoes on the skewers.

4. Place these skewers in an air fryer basket.

5. Press the "power button" of the air fry oven and turn the dial to select the "air fry" mode.

6. Press the time button and again turn the dial to set the cooking time to 25 minutes.

7. Now push the temp button and rotate the dial to set the temperature at 350 degrees f.

8. Once preheated, place the air fryer basket in the oven and close its lid.

9. Flip the skewers when cooked halfway through, then resume cooking.

10. Serve warm.

## 39. Yogurt Beef Kebabs

Preparation time: 10 minutes

Cooking time: 25 minutes

Servings: 4

**Ingredients:**

- ½ cup yogurt
- 1½ tablespoon mint
- 1 teaspoon ground cumin
- 1 cup eggplant, diced
- 10.5 oz. Lean beef, diced
- ½ small onion, cubed

**Directions:**

1. Whisk yogurt with mint and cumin in a suitable bowl.

2. Toss in beef cubes and mix well to coat. Marinate for 30 minutes.

3. Alternatively, thread the beef, onion, and eggplant on the skewers.

4. Place these beef skewers in the air fry basket.

5. Press the "power button" of the air fry oven and turn the dial to select the "air fryer" mode.

6. Press the time button and again turn the dial to set the cooking time to 25 minutes.

7. Now push the temp button and rotate the dial to set the temperature at 370 degrees f.

8. Once preheated, place the air fryer basket in the oven and close its lid.

9. Flip the skewers when cooked halfway through, then resume cooking.

10. Serve warm.

**40. Agave Beef Kebabs**

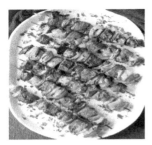

Preparation time: 10 minutes

Cooking time: 20 minutes

Servings: 6

**Ingredients:**

- 2 lbs. Beef steaks, cubed
- Two tablespoon jerk seasoning
- Zest and juice of 1 lime
- 1 tablespoon agave syrup
- ½ teaspoon thyme leaves, chopped

**Directions:**

1. Mix beef with jerk seasoning, lime juice, zest, agave and thyme.
2. Toss well to coat, then marinate for 30 minutes.
3. Alternatively, thread the beef on the skewers.
4. Place these beef skewers in the air fry basket.
5. Press the "power button" of the air fry oven and turn the dial to select the "air fryer" mode.
6. Press the time button and again turn the dial to set the cooking time to 20 minutes.
7. Now push the temp button and rotate the dial to set the temperature at 360 degrees f.
8. Once preheated, place the air fryer basket in the oven and close its lid.
9. Flip the skewers when cooked halfway through, then resume cooking.
10. Serve warm.

**41.Beef Skewers with Potato Salad**

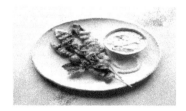

Preparation time: 10 minutes

Cooking time: 25 minutes

Servings: 4

**Ingredients:**

- Juice ½ lemon
- 2 tablespoon olive oil
- 1 garlic clove, crushed
- 1 ¼ lb. Diced beef
- For the salad
- 2 potatoes, boiled, peeled and diced
- 4 large tomatoes, chopped
- 1 cucumber, chopped
- 1 handful black olives, chopped
- 9 oz. Pack feta cheese, crumbled
- 1 bunch of mint, chopped

**Directions:**

1. Whisk lemon juice with garlic and olive oil in a bowl.
2. Toss in beef cubes and mix well to coat. Marinate for 30 minutes.
3. Alternatively, thread the beef on the skewers.
4. Place these beef skewers in the air fry basket.
5. Press the "power button" of the air fry oven and turn the dial to select the "air fryer" mode.
66. Press the time button and again turn the dial to set the cooking time to 25 minutes.
67. Now push the temp button and rotate the dial to set the temperature at 360 degrees f.
68. Once preheated, place the air fryer basket in the oven and close its lid.

69. Flip the skewers when cooked halfway through, then resume cooking.

70. Meanwhile, whisk all the salad ingredients in a salad bowl.

71. Serve the skewers with prepared salad.

## 42. Classic Souvlaki Kebobs

Preparation time: 10 minutes

Cooking time: 20 minutes

Servings: 6

**Ingredients:**

- 2 ¼ lbs. Beef shoulder fat trimmed, cut into chunks
- 1/3 cup olive oil
- ½ cup red wine
- 2 teaspoon dried oregano
- ½ cup of orange juice
- 1 teaspoon orange zest
- 2 garlic cloves, crushed

**Directions:**

1. Whisk olive oil, red wine, oregano, oranges juice, zest, and garlic in a suitable bowl.

2. Toss in beef cubes and mix well to coat. Marinate for 30 minutes.

3. Alternatively, thread the beef, onion, and bread on the skewers.

4. Place these beef skewers in the air fry basket.

5. Press the "power button" of the air fry oven and turn the dial to select the "air fryer" mode.

6. Press the time button and again turn the dial to set the cooking time to 20 minutes.

7. Now push the temp button and rotate the dial to set the temperature at 370 degrees f.

8. Once preheated, place the air fryer basket in the oven and close its lid.

9. Flip the skewers when cooked halfway through, then resume cooking.

10. Serve warm.

### 43. Harissa Dipped Beef Skewers

Preparation time: 10 minutes

Cooking time: 16 minutes

Servings: 6

**Ingredients:**

- 1 lb. Beef mince
- 4 tablespoon harissa
- 2 oz. Feta cheese
- One large red onion, shredded
- 1 handful parsley, chopped
- 1 handful mint, chopped
- 1 tablespoon olive oil
- Juice 1 lemon

**Directions:**

1. Whisk the lean beef in a bowl of harissa, onion, feta, and seasoning.

2. From this mixture, make 12 sausages, then thread them onto the skewers.

3. In the air-fry basket, put these beef skewers.

4. Click the Air Fry Oven control button and switch the knob to pick the bake mode.

5. To set the cooking time to 16 minutes, press the time button and turn the knob over again.

6. Now press the temp button to set the temperature at 370 degrees f and rotate the dial.

7. Place the air fryer basket in the oven until pre-heated and close the lid.

8. When done, rotate the skewers halfway through and then start cooking.

9. In a salad bowl, toss the remaining salad ingredients together.

10. Using tomato salad to eat beef skewers.

## 44. Onion Pepper Beef Kebobs

Preparation time: 10 minutes

Cooking time: 20 minutes

Servings: 4

**Ingredients:**

- 2 tablespoon pesto paste
- 2/3 lb. Beefsteak, diced
- 2 red peppers, cut into chunks
- 2 red onions, cut into wedges
- 1 tablespoon olive oil

**Directions:**

1. Toss the harissa and oil into the beef balls, then blend well to coat. For 30 minutes, marinate.

2. Thread the beef, onion, and peppers on the skewers as an option.

3. In the air-fry basket, put these beef skewers.

4. Click the air fryer's "power button" and change the knob to choose "air fryer" mode.

5. To set the cooking time to 20 minutes, click the time button and change the dial once again.

6. Now press the temp button to set the temperature at 370 degrees f and rotate the dial.

7. Place the air fryer basket in the oven until pre-heated and close the lid.

8. When done, rotate the skewers halfway through and then start cooking.

9. Serve it hot.

## 45.Mayo Spiced Kebobs

Preparation time: 10 minutes

Cooking time: 10 minutes

Servings: 4

**Ingredients:**

- 2 tablespoon cumin seed
- 2 tablespoon coriander seed
- 2 tablespoon fennel seed
- 1 tablespoon paprika
- 2 tablespoon garlic mayonnaise
- 4 garlic cloves, finely minced
- ½ teaspoon ground cinnamon
- 1 ½ lb. Lean minced beef

**Directions:**

1. Blend all the spices and seeds with garlic, cream, and cinnamon in a blender.

2. Add this cream paste to the minced beef, then mix well.

3. Make 8 sausages and thread each on the skewers.

4. Place these beef skewers in the air fry basket.

5. Press the "power button" of the air fry oven and turn the dial to select the "air fryer" mode.

6. Press the time button and again turn the dial to set the cooking time to 10 minutes.

7. Now push the temp button and rotate the dial to set the temperature at 370 degrees f.

8. Once preheated, place the air fryer basket in the oven and close its lid.

9. Flip the skewers when cooked halfway through, then resume cooking.

10. Serve warm.

### 46.Beef with Orzo Salad

Preparation time: 10 minutes

Cooking time: 27 minutes

Servings: 4

**Ingredients:**

- 2/3 lbs. Beef shoulder, cubed
- 1 teaspoon ground cumin
- ½ teaspoon cayenne pepper
- 1 teaspoon sweet smoked paprika
- 1 tablespoon olive oil
- 24 cherry tomatoes
- Salad:
- ½ cup orzo, boiled
- ½ cup frozen pea
- 1 large carrot, grated
- Small pack coriander, chopped
- Small pack mint, chopped
- Juice 1 lemon
- 2 tablespoon olive oil

**Directions:**

1. Toss tomatoes and beef with oil, paprika, pepper, and cumin in a bowl.

2. Alternatively, thread the beef and tomatoes on the skewers.

3. Place these beef skewers in the air fry basket.

4. Press the "power button" of the air fry oven and turn the dial to select the "air fryer" mode.

5. Press the time button and again turn the dial to set the cooking time to 25 minutes.

6. Now push the temp button and rotate the dial to set the temperature at 370 degrees f.

7. Once preheated, place the air fryer basket in the oven and close its lid.

8. Flip the skewers when cooked halfway through, then resume cooking.

9. Meanwhile, sauté carrots and peas with olive oil in a pan for 2 minutes.

10. Stir in mint, lemon juice, coriander, and cooked couscous.

11. Serve skewers with the couscous salad.

## 47.Beef Zucchini Shashliks

Preparation time: 10 minutes

Cooking time: 25 minutes

Servings: 4

**Ingredients:**

- 1lb. Beef, boned and diced
- 1 lime, juiced and chopped
- 3 tablespoon olive oil
- 20 garlic cloves, chopped
- 1 handful rosemary, chopped
- 3 green peppers, cubed

- 2 zucchinis, cubed
- 2 red onions, cut into wedges

**Directions:**

1. Toss the beef with the rest of the skewer's ingredients in a bowl.
2. Thread the beef, peppers, zucchini, and onion on the skewers.
3. Place these beef skewers in the air fry basket.
4. Press the "power button" of the air fry oven and turn the dial to select the "air fryer" mode.
5. Press the time button and again turn the dial to set the cooking time to 25 minutes.
6. Now push the temp button and rotate the dial to set the temperature at 370 degrees f.
7. Once preheated, place the air fryer basket in the oven and close its lid.
8. Flip the skewers when cooked halfway through, then resume cooking.
9. Serve warm.

## 48. Delicious Zucchini Mix

Total time: 25 min

Prep time: 10 min

Cook time: 15 min

Yield: 6 servings

**Ingredients:**

- 6 zucchinis, halved and then sliced
- Salt and black pepper to the taste
- 1 tablespoon of butter
- 1 teaspoon of oregano, dried
- ½ cup yellow onion, chopped
- 3 garlic cloves, minced

- 2 ounces of parmesan, grated
- ¾ cup of heavy cream

Directions:

1. On medium-high prepare, heat a saucepan that suits the butter of your Air Fryer, add onion, stir and cook for 4 minutes.

2. Mix the garlic, zucchini, oregano, salt, pepper and heavy cream together, shake, fry in the air and boil at 350 degrees F for 10 minutes.

3. Stir in the parmesan cheese, whisk, split and eat.

### 49.Swiss Chard and Sausage

Total time: 30 min

Prep time: 10 min

Cook time: 25 min

Yield: 8 servings

**Ingredients:**

- 8 cups of Swiss chard, chopped
- ½ cup of onion, chopped
- 1 tablespoon of olive oil
- 1 garlic clove, minced
- Salt and black pepper to the taste
- 3 eggs
- 2 cups of ricotta cheese
- 1 cup of mozzarella, shredded
- A pinch of nutmeg
- ¼ cup of parmesan, grated
- 1-pound sausage, chopped

**Directions:**

1. Heat up the Air Fryer with a saucepan that suits the oil over medium heat, add onions, garlic, Swiss chard, salt, pepper and nutmeg, stir, cook and turn off for 2 minutes.

2. In a bowl of mozzarella, parmesan, ricotta, whisk the eggs, stir, spillover Swiss chard blend, shake, put in your Air Fryer and cook at 320 °F for 17 minutes.

3. Divide and consume between bowls.

## 50. Swiss Chard Salad

Total time: 18 min

Prep time: 5 min

Cook time: 10 min

Yield: 4 servings

### Ingredients:

- 1 bunch of Swiss chard, torn
- 2 tablespoons of olive oil
- 1 small yellow onion, chopped
- A pinch of red pepper flakes
- ¼ cup of pine nuts, toasted
- ¼ cup of raisins
- 1 tablespoon of balsamic vinegar
- Salt and black pepper to the taste

### Directions:

1. Heat a medium-hot saucepan that fits the oil with your Air Fryer, add the chard and onions, stir and cook for 5 minutes.

2. Add the salt, pepper, pepper flakes, raisins, pine nuts and vinegar, stir, fry and simmer at 350 degrees F. for 8 minutes.

3. Divide and consume between bowls.

## 51. Spanish Greens

Total time: 18 min

Prep time: 5 min

Cook time: 10 min

Yield: 4 servings

**Ingredients:**

- 1 apple, cored and chopped
- 1 yellow onion, sliced
- 3 tablespoons of olive oil
- ¼ cup of raisins
- 6 garlic cloves, chopped
- ¼ cup of pine nuts, toasted
- ¼ cup of balsamic vinegar
- 5 cups of mixed spinach and chard
- Salt and black pepper to the taste
- A pinch of nutmeg

**Directions:**

1. Over medium-high pressure, heat a saucepan that fits the oil with your Air Fryer, add onion, stir and cook for 3 minutes.
2. Add the onion, ginger, raisins, sugar, mixed spinach, chard, nutmeg, salt and pepper, stir, and roast for 5 minutes at 350 degrees F.
3. Brush on top, break into bowls and serve with pine nuts.

**52.Flavored Air Fried Tomatoes**

Total time: 25 min

Prep time: 10 min

Cook time: 15 min

Yield: 6 servings

**Ingredients:**

- 1 jalapeno pepper, chopped

- 4 garlic cloves, minced
- 2 pounds of cherry tomatoes, halved
- Salt and black pepper to the taste
- ¼ cup of olive oil
- ½ teaspoon of oregano, dried
- ¼ cup of basil, chopped
- ½ cup of parmesan, grated

**Directions:**

1. In a cup, add the tomatoes with garlic, jalapeno, season with salt, pepper and oregano, drizzle with the oil, blend to cover, put in your Air Fryer and cook at 380 °F for 15 minutes.
2. Move the tomatoes to a pan, add the basil and parmesan, toss and eat.

**53. Italian Eggplant Stew**

Total time: 25 min

Prep time: 10 min

Cook time: 15 min

Yield: 6 servings

**Ingredients:**

- 1 red onion, chopped
- 2 garlic cloves, chopped
- 1 bunch of parsley, chopped
- Salt and black pepper to the taste
- 1 teaspoon of oregano, dried
- 2 eggplants, cut into medium chunks
- 2 tablespoons of olive oil
- 2 tablespoons of capers, chopped
- 1 handful green olives, pitted and sliced

- 5 tomatoes, chopped
- 3 tablespoons of herb vinegar

**Directions:**

1. Heat a medium-hot saucepan that fits the oil of your Air Fryer, add the eggplant, oregano, salt, and pepper, stir and cook for 5 minutes.

2. Combine the garlic, onions, parsley, capers, olives, vinegar and tomatoes, stir, fry and prepare at 360 °F for 15 minutes.

3. Break and serve in pots.

## 54. Rutabaga and Cherry Tomatoes Mix

Total time: 25 min

Prep time: 10 min

Cook time: 15 min

Yield: 6 servings

**Ingredients:**

- 1 tablespoon of shallot, chopped
- 1 garlic clove, minced
- ¾ cup of cashews, soaked for a couple of hours and drained
- 2 tablespoons of nutritional yeast
- ½ cup of veggie stock
- Salt and black pepper to the taste
- 2 teaspoons of lemon juice

**For the pasta:**

- 1 cup of cherry tomatoes, halved
- 5 teaspoons of olive oil
- ¼ teaspoon of garlic powder
- 2 rutabagas, peeled and cut into thick noodles

**Directions:**

1. Heat a medium-hot saucepan that fits the oil of your Air Fryer, add the eggplant, oregano, salt, and pepper, stir and cook for 5 minutes.

2. Combine the garlic, onions, parsley, capers, olives, vinegar and tomatoes, stir, fry and prepare at 360 °F for 15 minutes.

3. Break and serve in pots.

## 55. Garlic Tomatoes

Total time: 25 min

Prep time: 10 min

Cook time: 15 min

Yield: 6 servings

**Ingredients:**

- 4 garlic cloves, crushed
- 1-pound mixed cherry tomatoes
- 3 thyme springs, chopped
- Salt and black pepper to the taste
- ¼ cup of olive oil

**Directions:**

1. In a bowl of salt, black pepper, garlic, olive oil and thyme, mix the tomatoes, brush, place in the Air Fryer, and cook at 360 °F for 15 minutes.

2. Divide the tomatoes into bowls and serve.

## 56. Tomato and Basil Tart

Total time: 25 min

Prep time: 10 min

Cook time: 15 min

Yield: 6 servings

**Ingredients:**

- 1 bunch of basil, chopped

- 4 eggs
- 1 garlic clove, minced
- Salt and black pepper to the taste
- ½ cup of cherry tomatoes halved
- ¼ cup of cheddar cheese, grated

**Directions:**

1. In a cup, combine the eggs with the cinnamon, black pepper, cheese and basil, then whisk together well.

2. Place the tomatoes on top, put in the fryer, and cook at 320 ° F for 14 minutes in a baking dish that fits with your Air Fryer.

3. Cut on and serve.

4.

## 57. Zucchini Noodles Delight

Total time: 30 min

Prep time: 10 min

Cook time: 25 min

Yield: 6 servings

**Ingredients:**

- 2 tablespoons of olive oil
- 3 zucchinis, cut with a spiralizer
- 16 ounces of mushrooms, sliced
- ¼ cup sun-dried tomatoes, chopped
- 1 teaspoon of garlic, minced
- ½ cup of cherry tomatoes halved
- 2 cups of tomatoes sauce
- 2 cups of spinach, torn
- Salt and black pepper to the taste
- A bunch of basil, chopped

**Directions:**

1. In a bowl, place the zucchini noodles, season with salt and black pepper and leave for about 10 minutes.
2. Over medium-high heat, heat a pan that matches the oil with your Air Fryer, add the garlic, stir and cook for 1 minute.
3. Stir in mushrooms, sun-dried tomatoes, cherry tomatoes, spinach, cayenne, sauce, zucchini noodles, place in the Air Fryer, and cook at 320 degrees F for 10 minutes.
4. With sprinkled basil, divide between plates and pour-over.

## 58. Simple Tomatoes and Bell Pepper Sauce

Total time: 25 min

Prep time: 10 min

Cook time: 15 min

Yield: 6 servings

**Ingredients:**

- 2 red bell peppers, chopped
- 2 garlic cloves, minced
- 1-pound cherry tomatoes halved
- 1 teaspoon of rosemary, dried
- 3 bay leaves
- 2 tablespoons of olive oil
- 1 tablespoon of balsamic vinegar
- Salt and black pepper to the taste

**Directions:**

1. In a bowl, mix the tomatoes with the garlic, the salt, the black pepper, the rosemary, the bay leaves, half the oil, half the vinegar, and brush, and place in the Air Fryer and cook at 320 degrees F. for 15 minutes.

2. Meanwhile, in your food processor, mix the bell peppers with a touch of sea salt, black pepper, the rest of the oil, and the rest of the vinegar and mix very well.

3. Divide the roasted tomatoes into bowls, sauce them with the bell peppers and eat them.

### 59.Salmon with Thyme & Mustard

Preparation Time: 10 Minutes

Cooking Time: 10 Minutes

Servings: 2

**Ingredients:**

- 2 salmon fillets
- Salt and pepper to taste

- ½ teaspoon dried thyme

- 2 tablespoons mustard

- 2 teaspoons olive oil

- 1 clove garlic, minced

- 1 tablespoon brown sugar

## Directions:

1. Sprinkle salt and pepper on both sides of the salmon.

2. In a bowl, combine the remaining ingredients.

3. Spread this mixture on top of the salmon.

4. Place the salmon in the air fryer.

5. Choose the air fry function.

6. Cook at 400 degrees F for 10 minutes.

## 60. Lemon Garlic Fish Fillet

Preparation Time: 10 Minutes

Cooking Time: 30 Minutes

Servings: 2-4

## Ingredients:

- 2 white fish fillets

- Cooking spray

- ½ teaspoon lemon pepper

- ½ teaspoon garlic powder

- Salt and pepper to taste

- 2 teaspoon lemon juice

## Directions:

1. Choose a bake setting in your air fryer oven.

2. Preheat it to 360 degrees F.

3. Spray fish fillets with oil.

4. Season fish fillets with lemon pepper, garlic powder, salt and pepper.

5. Add to the air fryer.

6. Cook at 360 degrees F for 20 minutes.

7. Drizzle with lemon juice.

### 61.Blackened Tilapia

Preparation Time: 10 Minutes

Cooking Time: 35 Minutes

Servings: 4

**Ingredients:**

- 4 tilapia fillets
- Cooking spray
- 2 teaspoons brown sugar
- 2 tablespoons paprika
- ¼ teaspoon cayenne pepper
- 1 teaspoon garlic powder
- 1 teaspoon dried oregano
- ½ teaspoon cumin
- Salt to taste

**Directions:**

1. Spray fish fillets with oil.

2. Mix the remaining ingredients in a bowl.

3. Sprinkle both sides of fish with spice mixture.

4. Add to the air fryer.

5. Set it to air fry.

6. Cook at 400 degrees F for 4 to 5 minutes per side.

### 62.Fish & Sweet Potato Chips

Preparation Time: 10 Minutes

Cooking Time: 35 Minutes

Servings: 4

**Ingredients:**

- 4 cups sweet potatoes, sliced into strips
- 1 teaspoon olive oil
- 1 egg, beaten
- 2/3 cup breadcrumbs
- 1 teaspoon lemon zest
- 2 fish fillets, sliced into strips
- ½ cup Greek yogurt
- 1 tablespoon shallots, chopped
- 1 tablespoon chives, chopped
- 2 teaspoons dill, chopped

**Directions:**

1. Toss in the oil with the sweet potatoes.

2. Cook in an air fryer for 10 minutes or until crispy at 360 degrees F.

3. Just put aside.

4. Dip the fish fillet into your egg.

5. Dredge with lemon zest mixed with breadcrumbs.

6. Fry for 12 minutes at 360 degrees F.

7. Mix the milk along with the remaining ingredients.

8. Serve with fish, sweet potato chips, and sauce.

**63.Brussels Sprout Chips**

Preparation Time: 10 Minutes

Cooking Time: 15 Minutes

Servings: 2

**Ingredients:**

- 2 cups Brussels sprouts, sliced thinly
- 1 tablespoon olive oil
- 1 teaspoon garlic powder
- Salt and pepper to taste
- 2 tablespoons Parmesan cheese, grated

**Directions:**

1. In the oil, throw the Brussels sprouts.

2. Sprinkle the garlic, salt, pepper and Parmesan cheese with the garlic powder.

3. Select the Bake function.

4. In an air fryer, add the Brussels sprouts.

5. Cook for 8 minutes at 350 degrees F.

6. Flip and cook for an additional 7 minutes.

## 64. Shrimp Spring Rolls with Sweet Chili Sauce

Preparation Time: 10 Minutes

Cooking Time: 30 Minutes

Servings: 4

**Ingredients:**

- 2 ½ tbsp... sesame oil, divided
- 1 cup julienne-cut red bell pepper
- 1 cup matchstick carrots
- 2 cups pre-shredded cabbage
- ¼ cup chopped fresh cilantro
- 2 tsp. fish sauce
- ¼ tsp. crushed red pepper
- 1 tbsp... fresh lime juice
- ¾ cup julienne-cut snow peas
- 4 oz. peeled, deveined raw shrimp, chopped

- 8 (8-inch-square) spring roll wrappers
- ½ cup sweet chili sauce

**Directions:**

1. Pour in 1.5 teaspoons of the oil and let it heat over high heat until it smokes slightly. Get a big skillet. Toss the bell pepper, carrots, and cabbage in it now. Allow it to cook until the mixture is lightly wilted when constantly stirring (this takes 1 or 1.5 minutes). Spread on a rimmed baking sheet and leave for 5 minutes to cool.

2. Combine the cilantro, fish sauce, crushed red pepper, lime juice, snow peas, crabs, and a mixture of cabbage in a large bowl. Lightly stir.

3. Place on the work surface the spring roll wrappers so that you are facing one corner. Shift 1/4 cup of filling into the center of each spring roll wrapper using your spoon, while spreading it from left to right and into a 3-inch-long strip.

4. While tucking the tip of the corner under the filling, fold the bottom corner of each wrapper over the filling. Fold the left and right corners over the filling. Using water, lightly brush the remaining corner and roll the filled end of the wrapper into the remaining corner. Lastly, click to close softly. Dust two teaspoons of oil with the unused spring rolls.

5. In the air fryer basket, transfer the first four spring rolls and allow them to cook at 390 ° F for about 7 minutes. Flip the spring rolls after the first five minutes. For the other spring rolls, do the same.

6. Serve alongside spicy beef sauce with the cooked spring rolls.

**65.Coconut Shrimp and Apricot**

Preparation Time: 5 Minutes

Cooking Time: 35 Minutes

Servings: 6

**Ingredients:**

- 1-1/2 lbs. large shrimp, uncooked
- 1-1/2 cups sweetened shredded coconut
- ½ cup panko bread crumbs

- 4 large egg whites
- ¼ tsp. salt
- ¼ tsp. ground black pepper
- 3 dashes Louisiana-style hot sauce
- ½ cup all-purpose flour
- Cooking spray

## Sauce:

- 1 cup apricot preserves
- ¼ tsp. crushed red pepper flakes
- 1 tsp. cider vinegar

## Directions:

1. Make sure the air fryer is preheated to 375 F.

2. Peel the shrimp, eliminate the veins, but leave the tails.

3. Pick a shallow bowl and combine the coconut and breadcrumbs together.

4. Whisk the egg whites, salt, pepper, and hot sauce into another small mug.

5. Take up a third small bowl and place the flour in it.

6. To lightly coat, dip the shrimp into the flour. Through shaking, remove any excess flour.

7. In the egg white mixture and then in the coconut mixture, dip the flour-coated shrimp. Pat to ensure the compliance of the coating.

8. Spray the basket with cooking spray in your air fryer. If required, you can work in batches.

9. In the air fryer basket, arrange the shrimps so that they form a single plate.

10. Allow them to cook for 4 minutes. Turn the shrimp to the other side and cook until the coconut is finely browned and the shrimp is pink (this takes about 4 minutes).

11. Take a small saucepan when cooking the shrimps and mix the sauce ingredients in it. Then cook and whisk the mixture until the preserves are melted over medium-low heat.

12. Alongside the freshly cooked shrimps, serve the sauce.

## 66. Coconut Shrimp and Lime Juice

Preparation Time: 5 Minutes

Cooking Time: 30 Minutes

Servings: 4

**Ingredients:**

- 1½ tsp. black pepper
- ½ cup all-purpose flour
- 2 large eggs
- 2/3 cup unsweetened flaked coconut
- 1/3 cup panko (Japanese-style breadcrumbs)
- 12 oz. medium peeled, deveined raw shrimp, tail-on (about 24 shrimp)
- Cooking spray
- ½ tsp. kosher salt

**Sauce:**

- ¼ cup lime juice
- 1 serrano chile, thinly sliced
- ¼ cup honey
- 2 tsp. chopped fresh cilantro (optional)

**Directions:**

1. Get a shallow dish – and make a mixture of the pepper and the flour.

2. In a second shallow dish, beat the eggs.

3. Get a third shallow dish and mix the coconut and panko in it.

4. Hold each shrimp by the tail and dip into the flour mixture without coating the tail. Shake to get rid of the excess flour.

5. Dip in the egg mixture and allow any excess to drip off.

6. Finally, dip in the coconut mixture and press to ensure adherence.

7. Coat the shrimp generously with the cooking spray.

8. Transfer half of the shrimp to the air fryer basket and allow to cook for 6 to 8 minutes at 400 F.

9. Halfway into cooking, turn the shrimp to the other side and season with ¼ teaspoon of the salt.

10. Do the same for the other shrimps and salt also.

11. In the meantime, get a small bowl and whisk the lime juice, Serrano chile, and honey together.

12. Sprinkle the cooked shrimp with cilantro, and serve alongside the sauce (if desired).

## 67. Lemon Pepper Shrimp

Preparation Time: 5 Minutes

Cooking Time: 20 Minutes

Servings: 2

**Ingredients:**

- 1 lemon, juiced
- ¼ tsp. paprika
- ¼ tsp. garlic powder
- 1 tsp. lemon pepper
- 1 tbsp... olive oil
- 12 oz. uncooked medium shrimp, peeled and deveined
- 1 lemon, sliced

**Directions:**

1. Ensure that your air fryer is preheated to 400 F.

2. Make a mixture of lemon juice, paprika, garlic powder, lemon pepper, and olive oil in a bowl.

3. Toss in the shrimp and coat it with the mixture.

4. Transfer the shrimp into the air fryer and cook for about 8 minutes (until the shrimp is firm and pink).

5. Serve alongside lemon slices.

### 68. Air Fryer Shrimp Bang

Preparation Time: 10 Minutes

Cooking Time: 30 Minutes

Servings: 4

**Ingredients:**

- ¼ cup sweet chili sauce
- 1 tbsp... Sriracha sauce
- ½ cup mayonnaise
- ¼ cup all-purpose flour
- 1 cup panko bread crumbs
- 1 lb raw shrimp, peeled and deveined
- 1 head loose-leaf lettuce
- 2 green onions, chopped, or to taste (optional)

**Directions:**

1. Make sure the setting for your Air Fryer is 400 F.

2. In a bowl, produce a blend of garlic sauce, Sriracha sauce, and mayonnaise until a flat blend. If you like, hold a certain bang source aside in a separate dipping bowl.

3. Place on a plate the flour and on another plate the panko.

4. First, dip the shrimp into the rice, and then the paste of mayonnaise. Dip it into the panko, finally.

5. On a baking sheet, transfer the coated shrimp, then into the air fryer basket without overcrowding the basket.

6. Allow them to cook for 12 minutes.

7. For the remaining shrimp, do the same.

Serve the fried shrimp with green onions in lettuce wraps as a garnish.

## 69.Crispy Nachos Prawns

Preparation Time: 5 Minutes

Cooking Time: 20 Minutes

Servings: 6

**Ingredients:**

- 18 large prawns, peeled and deveined, tails left on

- 1 egg, beaten

- 1 (10 oz.) bag nacho-cheese flavored corn chips, finely crushed

**Directions:**

1. Rinse the prawns and dry by patting them.

2. Get a small bowl and whisk the egg in it. Transfer the crushed chips to a separate bowl.

3. Dip a prawn in the whisked egg and the crushed chips, respectively.

4. Transfer the coated prawn to a plate and do the same for the remaining prawns.

5. Ensure that your Air Fryer is preheated to 350 F.

6. Transfer the coated prawns into the air fryer and allow to cook for 8 minutes.

7. Opaque prawns mean they are well cooked.

8. Withdraw from the air fryer and serve.

## 70.Coconut Pumpkin Bars

Total time: 20 min

Prep time: 10 min

Cook time: 10 min

Yield: 12 serving

**Ingredients:**

- 2 eggs
- 1/4 cup coconut flour
- 8 oz. pumpkin puree
- 1/2 cup coconut oil, melted
- 1/3 cup swerve
- 1 1/2 tsp. pumpkin pie spice
- 1/2 tsp. baking soda
- 1 tsp. baking powder
- Pinch of salt

**Directions:**

1. Place the Cuisinart oven in place 1. with the rack.
2. Beat the eggs, coconut oil, pumpkin pie spice, sweetener, and pumpkin puree in a bowl until well mixed.
3. Mix the baking powder, coconut flour, salt, and baking soda together in another dish.
4. Apply the egg mixture to the coconut flour mixture and blend properly.
5. In the prepared baking pan, add the bar mixture in and spread evenly.
6. Set to bake for 33 minutes at 350 f. Place the baking dish in the preheated oven after five minutes.
7. Slice and serve.

**71. Almond Peanut Butter Bars**

Total time: 40 min

Prep time: 10 min

Cook time: 30 min

Yield: 8 serving

**Ingredients:**

- 2 eggs
- 1/2 cup erythritol
- 1/2 cup butter softened
- 1/2 cup peanut butter
- 1 tbsp. coconut flour
- 1/2 cup almond flour

**Directions:**

1. Place the cuisine-style oven with the rack in place 1.
2. Toss the honey, eggs, and peanut butter together in a bowl until well mixed.
3. Add the dried ingredients and mix until the batter is smooth.
4. Spread the batter in the greased baking pan evenly.
5. Set for 35 minutes to bake at 350 f. Place the baking sheet in the preheated oven after five minutes.
6. Cut and serve.

**72. Delicious Lemon Bars**

Total time: 40 min

Prep time: 10 min

Cook time: 30 min

Yield: 8 serving

**Ingredients:**

- 4 eggs
- 1 lemon zest
- 1/4 cup fresh lemon juice
- 1/2 cup butter softened
- 1/2 cup sour cream
- 1/3 cup erythritol

- 2 tsp. baking powder
- 2 cups almond flour

**Directions:**

1. Place the cuisine-style oven with the rack in place 1.
2. Whisk the eggs in a bowl until frothy.
3. Beat until well mixed, add butter and sour cream and beat.
4. Mix well with the sweetener, lemon zest, and lemon juice.
5. Add baking powder and almond flour and combine until mixed properly.
6. Move the batter and spread it evenly in a greased baking tray.
7. Set to bake for 45 minutes at 350 f. Place the baking sheet in the preheated oven after five minutes.
8. Cut and serve.

## 73. Easy Egg Custard

Total time: 50 min

Prep time: 10 min

Cook time: 40 min

Yield: 8 serving

**Ingredients:**

- 2 egg yolks
- 1 tsp. nutmeg
- 1/2 cup erythritol
- 2 cups heavy whipping cream
- 3 eggs
- 1/2 tsp. vanilla

**Directions:**

1. Place the Cuisinart oven in place 1. with the rack.

2. In the big mixing bowl, add all the ingredients and beat until just well mixed.

3. Pour the mixture of custard into the greased pie dish.

4. Set to bake for 40 minutes at 350 f. Place the pie dish in the preheated oven after five minutes.

5. Just serve.

**74.Flavors Pumpkin Custard**

Total time: 40 min

Prep time: 10 min

Cook time: 30 min

Yield: 8 serving

**Ingredients:**

- 4 egg yolks
- 1/2 tsp. cinnamon
- 1 tsp. liquid stevia
- 15 oz. pumpkin puree
- 3/4 cup coconut cream
- 1/8 tsp. cloves
- 1/8 tsp. ginger

**Directions:**

1. Place the cuisine-style oven with the rack in place 1.

2. Stir together the pumpkin puree, cloves, ginger, cinnamon, and swerve in a wide bowl.

3. Beat until well mixed, add egg yolks and beat.

4. Attach coconut cream and stir thoroughly.

5. Pour in the six ramekins with the mixture.

6. Set to bake for 45 minutes at 350 f. Place the ramekin in a preheated oven after 5 minutes.

7. Serve refrigerated and enjoy.

## 75. Almond Butter Cookies

Total time: 25 min

Prep time: 10 min

Cook time: 15 min

Yield: 15 serving

**Ingredients:**

- 1 egg
- 1/2 cup erythritol
- 1 cup almond butter
- 1 tsp. vanilla
- Pinch of salt

**Directions:**

1. Place the Cuisinart oven in place 1. with the rack.
2. In a big bowl, add all the ingredients and blend until well mixed.
3. Make cookies from the bowl mixture and put them on a baking pan lined with parchment.
4. Set for 20 minutes to bake at 350 f. Place the baking pan in the preheated oven after five minutes.
5. Just serve.

### 76.Tasty Pumpkin Cookies

Total time: 35 min

Prep time: 15 min

Cook time: 20 min

Yield: 8 serving

**Ingredients:**

- 1 egg
- 2 cups almond flour
- 1/2 tsp. baking powder
- 1 tsp. vanilla
- 1/2 cup butter
- 1 tsp. liquid stevia
- 1/2 tsp. pumpkin pie spice
- 1/2 cup pumpkin puree

**Directions:**

1. Place the Cuisinart oven in place 1. with the rack.
2. Put all the ingredients in a big bowl and blend until well mixed.
3. Make cookies from the mixture and put them on a baking sheet lined with parchment.
4. Set to bake for 30 minutes at 300 f. Place the baking dish in the preheated oven after five minutes.
5. Enjoy and serve.

6.

## 77.Almond Pecan Cookies

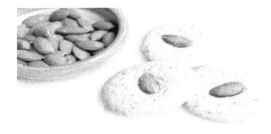

Total time: 30 min

Prep time: 10 min

Cook time: 20 min

Yield: 16 serving

**Ingredients:**

- 1/2 cup butter
- 1 tsp. vanilla
- 2 tsp. gelatin
- 2/3 cup swerve
- 1 cup pecans
- 1/3 cup coconut flour
- 1 cup almond flour

**Directions:**

1. Place the Cuisinart oven in place 1. with the rack.

2. In the food processor, add the butter, vanilla, gelatin, swerve, coconut flour, and almond flour and process until crumbs form.

3. Attach pecans and process them until they're chopped.

4. Make cookies from the prepared mixture and put them in a baking pan lined with parchment.

5. Set for 25 minutes to bake at 350 f. Place the baking pan in the preheated oven after five minutes.

6. Enjoy and serve.

## 78. Butter Cookies

Total time: 25 min

Prep time: 10 min

Cook time: 15 min

Yield: 24 serving

**Ingredients:**

- 1 egg, lightly beaten
- 1 tsp. vanilla
- 3/4 cup swerve
- 1 1/4 cups almond flour
- 1 tsp. baking powder
- 1 stick butter
- Pinch of salt

**Directions:**

1. Place the Cuisinart oven in place 1. with the rack.
2. Beat the butter and sweetener in a bowl until it is smooth.
3. Mix the almond flour and baking powder together in a separate dish.
4. Apply the butter mixture to the egg and vanilla and beat until smooth.
5. Apply the dry ingredients to the wet ingredients and stir until well mixed.
6. Cover the dough in plastic wrap and put it for 1 hour in the fridge.
7. Make cookies from the dough and put them on a baking sheet lined with parchment.
8. Set for 20 minutes to bake at 325 f. Place the baking pan in the preheated oven after five minutes.

9. Enjoy and serve.

## 79.Tasty Brownie Cookies

Total time: 30 min

Prep time: 10 min

Cook time: 20 min

Yield: 16 serving

### Ingredients:

- 1 egg
- 1/2 cup erythritol
- 1/4 cup cocoa powder
- 1 cup almond butter
- 3 tbsp. milk
- 1/4 cup chocolate chips

### Directions:

1. Place the Cuisinart oven in place 1. with the rack.
2. Mix the almond butter, egg, sweetener, almond milk, and cocoa powder together in a bowl until well mixed.
3. Stir in the crisps of Chocó.
4. Make cookies from the dough and put them on a baking sheet lined with parchment.
5. Set for 15 minutes to bake at 350 f. Place the baking pan in the preheated oven after five minutes.
6. Enjoy and serve.

## 80.Tasty Gingersnap Cookies

Total time: 20 min

Prep time: 10 min

Cook time: 10 min

Yield: 8 serving

**Ingredients:**

- 1 egg
- 1/2 tsp. ground cinnamon
- 1/2 tsp. ground ginger
- 1 tsp. baking powder
- 3/4 cup erythritol
- 1/2 tsp. vanilla
- 1/8 tsp. ground cloves
- 1/4 tsp. ground nutmeg
- 2/4 cup butter, melted
- 1 1/2 cups almond flour
- Pinch of salt

**Directions:**

1. Place the Cuisinart oven in place 1. with the rack.
2. Mix all the dried ingredients together in a mixing bowl.
3. Blend all the wet ingredients together in another tub.
4. Apply the dry ingredients to the wet ingredients and blend until the mixture is dough-like.
5. Cover and place for 30 minutes in the refrigerator.
6. Make cookies from the dough and put them on a baking sheet lined with parchment.
7. Set for 15 minutes to bake at 350 f. Place the baking pan in the preheated oven after five minutes.
8. Enjoy and serve.

### 81.Simple Lemon Pie

Total time: 55 min

Prep time: 25 min

Cook time: 30 min

Yield: 8 serving

**Ingredients:**

- 3 eggs
    - oz. butter, melted
- 3 lemon juice
- 1 lemon zest, grated
- 4 oz. erythritol
    - oz. almond flour
- Salt

**Directions:**

1. Place the cuisine-style oven with the rack in place 1.
2. Mix the butter, 1 oz. of sweetener, 3 oz. of almond flour, and salt together in a dish.
3. Move the dough to a pie dish and cook for 20 minutes, spreading uniformly.
4. Mix the eggs, lemon juice, lemon zest, remaining flour, sweetener and salt together in a separate dish.
5. Pour the mixture of eggs into a prepared crust.
6. Set for 35 minutes to bake at 350 f. Place the pie dish in the preheated oven after five minutes.
7. Cut and serve.

## 82. Flavorful Coconut Cake

Total time: 30 min

Prep time: 10 min

Cook time: 25 min

Yield: 10 servings

**Ingredients:**

- 5 eggs, separated

- 1/2 cup erythritol
- 1/4 cup coconut milk
- 1/2 cup coconut flour
- 1/2 tsp. baking powder
- 1/2 tsp. vanilla
- 1/2 cup butter softened
- Pinch of salt

**Directions:**

1. Place the cuisine-style oven with the rack in place 1.
2. Grease the buttered cake pan and set it aside.
3. Beat the sweetener and butter together in a bowl until mixed.
4. Mix well with the egg yolks, coconut milk, and vanilla.
5. Stir well and apply baking powder, coconut flour and salt.
6. Beat the egg whites in another bowl until a stiff peak emerges.
7. Fold the egg whites gently into the cake mixture.
8. In a prepared cake pan, pour batter into it.
9. Set to bake for 25 minutes at 400 f. Place the cake pans in the preheated oven for 5 minutes.
10. Cut and serve.

## 83. Easy Lemon Cheesecake

Total time: 55 min

Prep time: 10 min

Cook time: 35 min

Yield: 10 servings

**Ingredients:**

- 4 eggs
- 2 tbsp. swerve
- 1 fresh lemon juice

- 18 oz. ricotta cheese
- 1 fresh lemon zest

**Directions:**

1. Place the cuisine-style oven with the rack in place 1.
2. Beat the ricotta cheese in a large bowl until smooth.
3. Attach one egg at a time and whisk well.
4. Mix well with lemon juice, lemon zest, and swerve.
5. To the greased cake pan, move the mixture.
6. Set for 60 minutes to bake at 350 f. Place the cake pans in the preheated oven for 5 minutes.
7. Cut and serve.

**84. Lemon Butter Cake**

Total time: 55 min

Prep time: 20 min

Cook time: 35 min

Yield: 10 servings

**Ingredients:**

- 4 eggs
- 1/2 cup butter softened
- 2 tsp. baking powder
- 1/4 cup coconut flour
- 2 cups almond flour
- 2 tbsp. lemon zest
- 1/2 cup fresh lemon juice
- 1/4 cup erythritol
- 1 tbsp. vanilla

**Directions:**

1. Place the Cuisinart oven in place 1. with the rack.

2. Whisk all the ingredients in a wide bowl until a smooth batter is created.

3. Fill the loaf pan with butter.

4. Set to bake for 60 minutes at 300 f. Place the loaf pan in the preheated oven after five minutes.

5. Slicing and serving.

## 85. Cream Cheese Butter Cake

Total time: 45 min

Prep time: 10 min

Cook time: 35 min

Yield: 10 servings

### Ingredients:

- 5 eggs
- 1 cup swerve
- 4 oz. cream cheese, softened
- 1 tsp. vanilla
- 1 tsp. orange extract
- 1 tsp. baking powder
- oz. almond flour
- 1/2 cup butter, softened

### Directions:

1. Place the cuisine-style oven with the rack in place 1.

2. In the mixing bowl, add all the ingredients and whisk until fluffy.

3. Pour the batter into a cake pan that has been prepared.

4. Set for 40 minutes to bake at 350 f. Place the cake pans in the preheated oven for 5 minutes.

5. Slice and serve

## 86. Easy Ricotta Cake

Total time: 55 min

Prep time: 20 min

Cook time: 35 min

Yield: 8 servings

**Ingredients:**

- 2 eggs
- 1/2 cup erythritol
- 1/4 cup coconut flour
- 15 oz. ricotta
- Pinch of salt

**Directions:**

1. Place the cuisine-style oven with the rack in place 1.
2. Mix the eggs in a dish.
3. Connect the remaining ingredients and blend until well mixed.
4. Apply the batter to the greased cake tray.
5. Set to bake for 50 minutes at 350 f. Place the cake pans in the preheated oven for 5 minutes.
6. Cut and serve.

**87.Strawberry Muffins**

Total time: 45 min

Prep time: 10 min

Cook time: 35 min

Yield: 10 servings

**Ingredients:**

- 4 eggs
- 1/4 cup water
- 1/2 cup butter, melted
- 2 tsp. baking powder

- 2 cups almond flour
- 2/3 cup strawberries, chopped
- 2 tsp. vanilla
- 1/4 cup erythritol
- Pinch of salt

**Directions:**

1. Place the Cuisinart oven in place 1. with the rack.
2. Line and set aside 12-cups of a muffin tin with cupcake liners.
3. Mix the almond flour, baking powder, and salt together in a medium dish.
4. Whisk the eggs, sweetener, vanilla, water, and butter together in a separate cup.
5. Apply the mixture of almond flour to the egg mixture and stir until well mixed.
6. Attach the strawberries and stir thoroughly.
7. Pour the batter into the muffin tin that has been packed.
8. Set for 25 minutes to bake at 350 f. Place the muffin tin in the preheated oven for 5 minutes.
9. Enjoy and serve.

**88.Mini Brownie Muffins**

Total time: 35 min

Prep time: 10 min

Cook time: 25 min

Yield: 10 servings

**Ingredients:**

- 3 eggs
- 1/2 cup swerve
- 1 cup almond flour

- 1 tbsp. gelatin
- 1/3 cup butter, melted
- 1/3 cup cocoa powder

**Directions:**

1. Place the Cuisinart oven in place 1. with the rack.
2. Set aside and line 6-cups of a muffin tin with cupcake liners.
3. In the mixing bowl, add all ingredients and stir until well mixed.
4. In the prepared muffin pan, pour the mixture into it.
5. Set for 20 minutes to bake at 350 f. Place the muffin tin in the preheated oven for 5 minutes.
6. Enjoy and serve.

**89.Cinnamon Cheesecake Bars**

Total time: 35 min

Prep time: 10 min

Cook time: 25 min

Yield: 10 servings

**Ingredients:**

- Nonstick cooking spray
- 16 oz. Cream cheese, soft
- 1 tsp. vanilla
- 1 ¼ cups sugar, divided
- 2 tubes refrigerated crescent rolls
- 1 tsp. cinnamon
- ¼ cup butter

**Directions:**

1. Place the rack in position 1. Using cooking spray to spray the bottom of an 8x11-inch pan.

2. Beat the cream cheese, vanilla, and 3⁄4 cup sugar in a medium bowl until smooth.

3. On the bottom of the prepared pan, roll out one can of crescent rolls, close the perforations, and press the sides partway up.

4. Spread the mixture of cream cheese uniformly over the crescents.

5. Roll out the second can of crescents, covering the perforations over the top of the cheese mixture.

6. Stir the cinnamon and the remaining sugar together in a small cup. Let the butter melt.

7. Set the oven to 375 °F for 35 minutes to bake.

8. Sprinkle over the top of the crescents with the cinnamon sugar and drizzle with melted butter.

9. Place the pan in the oven after the oven has preheated for 5 minutes, then bake for 30 minutes until the top is golden brown.

10. Absolutely cool. Before slicing and serving, cover and refrigerate for at least 2 hours.

## 90. Strawberry Cobbler

Total time: 35 min

Prep time: 10 min

Cook time: 25 min

Yield: 10 servings

**Ingredients:**

- Butter flavored cooking spray
- 2 tbsp. Cornstarch
- ¼ cup fresh lemon juice
- ½ cup + 1 tbsp. Sugar divided
- 3 cups strawberries, hulled & sliced
- 5 tbsp. Butter, cold & diced

- 1 cup flour
- 1 ½ tsp. baking powder
- ½ tsp. salt
- ½ cup heavy cream

**Directions:**

1. Place the rack in position 1. Using cooking spray to spray a 9-inch baking pan.

2. Combine the cornstarch, lemon juice, and half a cup of sugar in a saucepan. Cook, constantly stirring, over medium heat, until the sugar dissolves and the mixture thickens.

3. Remove from the heat and stir in the berries gently. Pour 2 teaspoons of butter into a prepared pan and sprinkle.

4. Combine the flour, remaining sugar, baking powder, and salt in a large bowl. Split the remaining butter using a fork or pastry cutter until the mixture resembles coarse crumbs.

5. Stir in the cream and sprinkle the strawberries over them.

6. Set the oven to 400 degrees F for 30 minutes to bake. Place the cobbler in the oven after five minutes and bake for 25 minutes until bubbly and golden brown. Let cool 10 minutes prior to serving, at least.

**91.Baked Zucchini Fries**

Total time: 20 min

Prep time: 10 min

Cook time: 10 min

Yield:  4 servings

**Ingredients:**

- 3 medium zucchinis, sliced lengthwise
- 1/2 cup of
- 2 egg, the white part
- 1/4 teaspoon of garlic powder

- 2 tablespoons of parmesan cheese, grated
- Salt and pepper to taste

**Directions**

1. Whisk the egg whites together in a bowl and season with salt and pepper.

2. In a separate dish, combine the garlic powder, breadcrumbs, and cheese together.

3. Dip the zucchini sticks into one after the other of the egg, bread crumb and cheese mixture, then place the Air Fryer tray on a single layer.

4. Coat lightly with cooking spray and bake for about 15 minutes at 390 °F until golden brown.

5. Serve with a marinara sauce for dipping.

**92. Roasted Heirloom Tomato with Baked Feta**

Total time: 20 min

Prep time: 10 min

Cook time: 10 min

Yield: 4 servings

**Ingredients:**

**For the Tomato:**

- 2 heirloom tomatoes, sliced thickly into ½ inch circular slices
- 1 8-ounceof feta cheese, sliced thickly into ½ inch circular slices
- ½ cup of red onions, sliced thinly
- 1 pinch of salt
- 1 tablespoon of olive oil

**For the Basil Pesto:**

- ½ cup of basil, chopped roughly
- ½cup of parsley, roughly chopped
- 3 tablespoons of pine nuts, toasted

- ½ cup of parmesan cheese, grated
- 1 garlic clove
- 1 pinch of salt
- ½ cup of olive oil

**Directions:**

1. Start by making pesto. To do this, a food processor mixes garlic, parmesan, parsley, toasted pine nuts, basil, and salt.

2. Turn it on and eventually apply the olive oil to the pesto. Store and place in the refrigerator until finished, before ready to use.

3. Preheat the 390 ° F Air Fryer. Pat a dried tomato with a towel on paper. Spread a tablespoon of the pesto on top of each tomato slice and top with the feta. Add the red onions and toss with 1 tablespoon of olive oil; put on top of the feta.

4. In the cooking bowl, put the feta/ tomatoes and cook until the feta is brownish and begins to soften, or 12 to 14 minutes.

5. Add 1 spoonful of basil pesto and a tablespoon of salt. Enjoy and serve.

**93. Garam Masala Beans**

Total time: 20 min

Prep time: 10 min

Cook time: 10 min

Yield:  4 servings

**Ingredients:**

- 9-ounce of Beans
- 2 Eggs
- 1/2 cup of breadcrumbs
- 1/2 cup of flour
- 1/2 teaspoon of garam masala
- 2 teaspoon of chili powder

- Olive Oil
- Salt to taste

**Directions:**

1. At 350°F, preheat the Air Fryer. In a cup, combine the chili powder, garam masala, flour, and salt, and stir well. Place the eggs in one hand and beat them.

2. On a different pan, pour the breadcrumbs and then cover the beans with the flour mixture. Now dip the beans in the mixture of the eggs and then the breadcrumbs. For all the beans, do this.

3. Place the beans and cook for 4 minutes in the Air Fryer tray. Open and coat the oil on the beans and simmer again for another 3 minutes. Serve it hot.

### 94.Crisp Potato Wedges

Total time: 20 min

Prep time: 10 min

Cook time: 10 min

Yield:  4 servings

**Ingredients:**

- 3 teaspoons of olive oil
- 2 big potatoes
- ¼ cup of sweet chili sauce
- ¼ cup of sour cream

**Directions:**

1. To build a wedge shape, slice the potatoes lengthwise.

2. Hot the 356 ° F Air Fryer.

3. In a bowl, put the wedges and add the oil. Toss gently until the oil is thoroughly coated with the potatoes.

4. Place the side of the skin facing down into the cooking basket and cook for about 15 minutes. Toss, then cook until golden brown for another 10 minutes.

5. Best eaten with chili and sour cream when warm.

## 95.Crispy Onion Rings

Total time: 20 min

Prep time: 10 min

Cook time: 10 min

Yield:  4 servings

### Ingredients:

- 1 big of sized onion, thinly sliced
- 8 ounces of milk
- 1 egg
- 6 ounces of breadcrumbs
- 1 teaspoon of baking powder
- 10 ounces of flour
- 1teaspoon of salt

### Directions:

1. Heat your Air Fryer to 360°F for 10 minutes.

2. Detach the onion slices to separate rings.

3. Mix the baking powder, flour, and salt in a bowl.

4. Put the onion rings into the flour mixture to coat them. Beat the egg and the milk and stir into the flour to form a batter. Dip the flour-coated rings in the batter.

5. Put the breadcrumbs in a small tray, place the onion rings in it, and ensure all sides are well coated.

6. Place the rings in the fryer basket and air fry for 10 minutes until crisp.

## 96.Cheese Lasagna and Pumpkin Sauce

Total time: 20 min

Prep time: 10 min

Cook time: 10 min

Yield:  2 servings

**Ingredients:**

- 25 ounces of pumpkin, peeled and finely chopped
- 4 teaspoons of finely chopped rosemary
- 17½ ounces of beets, cooked and thinly sliced
- 1 medium-sized onion, chopped
- 1 cup of goat's cheese, grated
- Grana Padano cheese, grated
- 28 ounces of tomatoes, cubed
- 6 teaspoons of olive oil
- 8½ ounces of lasagna sheets

**Directions:**

1. In a cup, mix the pumpkin, 3 teaspoons of oil, and rosemary and fry for 10 minutes at 347 degrees F.

2. To mix the rosemary, peppers, and onions into a puree, remove the pumpkin from the Air Fryer and use a hand blender. In a saucepan, pour the puree and put it over low heat for 5 minutes.

3. Grease a dish that is heatproof with grease. First, put the pumpkin sauce and then the lasagna sheets in. Divide the sauce into two, and the goat cheese and beets into three. Put on the lasagna a portion of the beets and sauce and top with a portion of the goat cheese. Repeat this until all the ingredients are used, and you finish it with cheese and sauce.

4. Add the lasagna and air fried the Grana Padano at 300 ° F for 45 minutes. Detach and allow to cool.

5. Using a cookie cutter to cut out circular shapes and roast for 6 minutes at 390 ° F. Garnish with the goats' grated cheese and beet slices.

## 97.Pasta Wraps

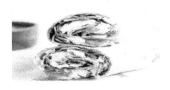

Total time: 20 min

Prep time: 10 min

Cook time: 10 min

Yield: 2 servings

**Ingredients:**

- 8 ounces of flour
- 2 ounces of pasta
- 6 teaspoons of olive oil
- 1clove of garlic, chopped
- 1 green chili, chopped
- 1 small onion, chopped
- 1tablespoon of tomato pastes
- ½ teaspoon of garam masala
- Salt to taste

**Directions:**

1. Mix the flour with water and salt to make a dough. Add 1teaspoon of the oil mixture and set aside.

2. Put the pasta in boiling water and add 3 teaspoons of oil and salt to it. Drain excess water when cooked.

3. Sauté the onions, garlic, chili, and add the spices, salt, and tomato paste. Lastly, add the cooked pasta and cover with a lid and turn down the heat to low.

4. Preheat the Air fryer to 390ºF.

5. Mold the dough into small balls; flatten them using a rolling pin into a circle. Put the pasta stuffing on them and fold the opposite edges together—seal edges with water.

6. Place into the Air Fryer and cook for 15 minutes until golden. Remove and serve while hot with a sauce.

## 98.Homemade Tater Tots

Total time: 20 min

Prep time: 10 min

Cook time: 10 min

Yield:  2 servings

**Ingredients:**

- 1 medium-sized russet potato, chopped

- 1 teaspoon of ground onion

- 1 teaspoon of vegetable oil

- ½ teaspoon of ground black pepper

- Salt to taste

**Directions:**

1. Boil the potatoes until they are a little more like al dente. Drain the water, add the onions, oil, and pepper and mash with the mixture.

2. Preheat the 379 º F Air Fryer.

3. Mold the potatoes into tater tots with the mash. Place the fryer in the air and bake for eight minutes. Shake the tots and bake for a further 5 minutes.

## 99.Mushroom, Onion, and Feta Frittata

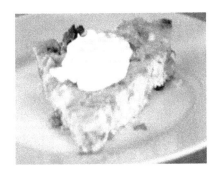

Total time: 20 min

Prep time: 10 min

Cook time: 10 min

Yield: 2 serving

**Ingredients:**

- 4 cups of button mushrooms, cleaned and cut thinly into¼ inch

- 6eggs

- 1 red onion, peeled and sliced thinly into¼ an inch

- 6 tablespoons of feta cheese, crumbled

- 2 tablespoons of olive oil

- 1 pinch of salt

**Directions**

1. In a sauté pan, apply the olive oil and swirl the onions and mushrooms about until tender under medium pressure. Remove from the heat on a dry kitchen towel and cool.

2. Preheat the 330°F Air Fryer. A touch of salt is added to whisk the eggs thoroughly in a mixing Bowland.

3. The inside and bottom of an 8-in suit. Slightly heat tolerant baking dish with mist. Through the baking bowl, pour the whisked eggs, apply the onion and mushroom mixture and then add the cheese.

4. Place the dish in the cooking basket and cook in the Air Fryer for 27 to 30 minutes or until a knife inserted in the middle of the frittata comes out clean.

## 100. Roasted Bell Pepper Vegetable Salad

Total time: 20 min

Prep time: 10 min

Cook time: 10 min

Yield: 2 serving

**Ingredients:**

- 1½ ounces of yogurt
- 1 medium-sized red bell pepper
- 2ounces of rocket leaves
- 3 teaspoons of lime juice
- 1 romaine lettuce
- 1 ounce of olive oil
- Ground black pepper and salt to taste

**Directions:**

1. Heat the Air-Fryer to 392 degrees F and put the bell pepper in it. Roast until a little charred for 10 minutes. Put the pepper in a dish, cover it, and leave for 15 minutes or so.

2. Divide the bell pepper into four parts, remove the skin and seeds and cut the pepper into thin strips.

3. In a bowl, carefully mix the lime juice, olive oil, and yogurt together. As needed, add the salt and pepper and stir.

4. Add the yogurt mixture to the rocket beans, broccoli, and pepper strips and toss to combine.

5.

## Conclusion

Air fryers are amazing both for food and health. This book is a compilation of amazing breakfast, lunch, meat, vegetarian, snack and dessert recipes that you can prepare at home using an air fryer and relish with your family.

CPSIA information can be obtained
at www.ICGtesting.com
Printed in the USA
BVHW061127040321
601715BV00006B/427